A MIND THAT FOUND ITSELF

A MIND THAT FOUND ITSELF

An Autobiography

CLIFFORD WHITTINGHAM BEERS

With a preface by Robert Coles

UNIVERSITY OF PITTSBURGH PRESS

Pittsburgh and London

Publication of this edition of
A Mind That Found Itself
was made possible by a grant from
the American Foundation for Mental Hygiene, Inc.

Published by the University of Pittsburgh Press, Pittsburgh, Pa., 15261, by
arrangement with Doubleday & Company, Inc.

Library of Congress Cataloging in Publication Data

Beers, Clifford Whittingham, 1876-1943.
    A mind that found itself.

    (Contemporary community health series)
    Reprint. Originally published: 5th ed. New York: Longmans, Green, 1921.
With new introd.
    1.   Psychiatric hospital care—United States—History.   2.   Beers,
Clifford Whittingham, 1876-1943.   3.   Mentally ill—United States—
Biography.   I.   Title.   II.   Series.
RC439.B4   1981   362.2'0973 [B]   80-5256
ISBN 0-8229-3442-6   AACR2
ISBN 0-8229-5324-2 (pbk.)

Dedicated
to the memory of my uncle
SAMUEL EDWIN MERWIN
whose timely generosity I believe saved my life,
and whose death has forever robbed
me of a satisfying opportunity
to prove my gratitude

Foreword

A Mind That Found Itself has been reprinted forty-one times since its publication in 1908.

Why is it that this volume continues to command the attention of the public after so many years? There are a number of reasons, and these become clear as one reads this fascinating and gripping autobiography of a man who suffered a severe mental illness, who recovered and set about to revolutionize and improve the care of the mentally ill both in this country and around the world.

A Mind That Found Itself is as engrossing today as when it burst upon the professional and the lay communities more than seventy years ago. The sense of shock is still there. The humanity, and the inhumanity, we feel as we live through this experience with Clifford Beers are profoundly depressing and inspiring at the same time. We are there at the birth of his concept of a national mass movement to prevent and to treat mental illness. This is Beers' great contribution to the American people, and the people of the world.

Clifford Beers must be counted as one of the mighty social reformers of the twentieth century. This book and a lifetime devoted to the development of community support for improved treatment and care, and for preventive services as well, have changed the course of our history.

But the great battle in which Beers engaged us when he organized the mental hygiene movement has not yet been won, even though substantial reforms and progress have been achieved. We must redouble our efforts to bring to fruition the great goals that Clifford Beers envisioned when he launched the mental hygiene movement.

William T. Beaty II, Secretary
American Foundation for Mental Hygiene, Inc.
1980

Preface

When William Carlos Williams was working on his autobiography, he paused occasionally to wonder about that particular medium of expression. To a young, aspiring doctor, he noted this in a letter: "We're all 'characters' in the big play—the story of our lives. I've been trying to step back from myself, but it's hard. Maybe it's wrong to do so. A lot of us are taught to be 'objective'; we lose ourselves that way. The trick is to *present* oneself—good and bad nature both. The trick is to remember that drama isn't only something you see on a stage or hear on a radio or read about. I am the novelist, I am the subject of the novel—some megalomania like that has to be in the bank account of a young writer, and even an old one has to have a few familiar 'acts' to fall back upon!"

All writers, Dr. Williams knew, call upon their own life for "material." He was, once again, acknowledging the intensely personal nature of his literary occupation—as always, with disarming candor. He understood that subjectivity could be thoughtful and contained; that self-description need not turn into self-indulgence, that psychology need not be the handmaiden of an imperial, categorical theory of psychopathology. Such knowledge, these days, cannot be taken for granted—not when anyone's humanity becomes a foil, so often, for those who wed a smug self-consciousness to a conviction that no one, anywhere, is to be let off this or that clinical or diagnostic hook.

Under such cultural circumstances, even to dare write an autobiography, never mind write the kind Clifford Beers wrote, is to take the obvious high risks—turn oneself into an occasion for various minds to have a day of it with their labels, their "explanations" for everything, their endlessly reductive arguments as to what causes what.

But Williams knew that literature—yes, even autobiography —must be judged on literary, on artistic merits. It won't do for us to regard *A Mind That Found Itself* as yet another example of the workings of a "psychotic process." Thousands upon thousands of deeply troubled and hurt men and women have, surely, tried to tell their stories—have written letters full of sadness, despair, self-justification, in the hope, thereby, that others would stop, read, pay heed, and finally, understand. But such writing, as those of us who have had to endure it know, prompts compassion (one hopes) and maybe a kind of clinical understanding, but not the larger response that a work of art commands—a broadened moral sensibility.

Without question *A Mind That Found Itself* is a work of art—a successful narrative worthy of inclusion in a tradition of intense, probing introspection. One thinks of St. Augustine's *Confessions,* of Rousseau's similarly titled personal expedition, of Freud's self-discovery *(Interpretation of Dreams),* of the inquiries into mental life achieved by de Quincey, by Rimbaud, and in this century, by Gertrude Stein or Dr. Williams or the young poets who followed his lead, the so-called beat ones with their dramatic departures from an accepted social and psychological morality. Clifford Beers was not the equal of such distinguished writers, but he wrote a decisively important essay on self, so to speak, and it entered the annals not only of successful autobiography (art), but American social history.

The very title of Beers' book tells us what helped him write it —a capacity for detachment, for wry, even ironic self-observation. Here is a man who wants to tell us about a serious bout with craziness, who invites our attention to his words with a phrase at once simple and dramatic, yet also impersonal, no matter that the most intimate matters of the human soul are to be laid bare. With each page, moreover, that almost uncanny mix of the title holds strong—a measure of distance, though at the same time an unflinching recital of one soul's anguish. We are captivated, really, by a writer who has mastered the art of composing strong, direct prose and who has found for himself a particular, commanding, enticing voice. No one, however scholarly and anxious to teach others, can win over a significant body of readers unless he or she, in some fashion, manages to persuade countless strangers that their time and attention will be well rewarded. In no time, Clifford Beers envelops us— a sincere, somewhat innocent young man, of solid but not especially elevated stock, who seems to have a reasonable number of good things going for him, but who suddenly feels upon his shoulder the strong, demanding, squeezing hand of fate.

It is a *story* we are told. A boy in a certain family suddenly becomes his brother's keeper—witness to the fateful tragedy of illness, and soon enough, caught up in a dreadful disaster all his own. Again, one notes how skillfully yet, it seems, with matter-of-fact naiveté, this tale of extreme woe unfolds. We are carried back to an earlier, small town America. We meet a given family. We sense their strength, their vulnerabilities. Trouble and more trouble accrue as our central character (the authorial presence, the narrator) pushes ahead in his account, and we know, in his life. He becomes a Yale undergraduate and graduate—an event of no small significance in his future life. That is to say, he enters the higher realms of class—and that was especially the case at the turn of the century. Then comes an aspiring business career. We seem on the brink of entering the New York world Edith Wharton documented, and in our time, Louis Auchincloss: money and influence obtained by those who have learned how to read good books, dress and

speak well, play certain sports—the power and the glory of the
Ivy League, Wall Street, fashionable East Coast upper-class
life.

One more ambitious, talented aspirant—and yet, Clifford
Beers would find his destiny, his celebrity, even his acquaintance with the rich and mighty world of American finance, in
quite another way. He stumbled right off, and for a while he
was headed nowhere fast. He introduces us to the experience
of mental illness with a storyteller's mastery of detail. It is, too,
a gradual and subtle introduction—one not apt to frighten us
away, or preclude further, persistent interest. Steadily, forth-
rightly, we come in touch with the nature of delusions and
hallucinations: the complex, symbolically charged, nightmarish
world of fear, suspicion, irritability and truculence—where any
word or gesture by anyone can become the catalytic instrument
of the fiercest of obsessions, antagonisms. The nature of paranoia—evidence of extreme self-preoccupation—has been portrayed acutely, suggestively, and unforgettably by Shakespeare
and Dostoevsky, by Kafka and Céline and Sartre; Beers is not
their peer, but he is no dull archivist of symptomatology, anxious for us to memorize a given list in preparation for an examination. He provides the virtues of clinical analysis, as well as
personal reminiscence, all rendered with a novelist's eye for the
particular, for emotional nuance, for chronological progression.
The applause this book received from writers such as Booth
Tarkington and William James has to do not only with its
important, knowing factuality, but with its especially winning
and convincing mode of presentation.

And again, the drama: a psychotic patient moves from the
isolation, the brooding silence, the shut off anguish of a certain
kind of paranoia to the giddy, talkative, all too energetic exuberance of manic ascension—a shift of gears which can't help
but keep the reader's attention, and not out of sadistic voyeur-
ism, one hastens to add, but as a response to a compelling shift

in a story's course of action. Nor is the issue only psychiatric—a "case" developing along certain clinical lines. This was a layman, writing almost a century ago; yet, he was utterly up to date, so far as our present thinking goes, on the nature of mental illness and the correct approach to its treatment. Beers knew, before Freud's writing had become part of our culture, that symptoms are connected to earlier life experiences; and that the treatment of those symptoms will, inevitably, vary a great deal—by virtue of one's "class and caste," one's place of residence, one's education, one's "background," as it is sometimes put.

What A. B. Hollingshead and F. C. Redlich documented in Connecticut during the 1950s and wrote up as *Social Class and Mental Illness,* Clifford Beers had explored and also written up, after his own fashion: an earlier Connecticut, an earlier America—then, as now, not able to separate altogether successfully medical need and availability from personal or familial social position. As Beers descended into illness, he and his family lost their economic resources. The consequences were all too quickly forthcoming—worse and worse medical care. This is a muckraking book, and alas, the aptness of the polemic is still to be remarked upon. I have in my own professional career, as a child psychiatrist, seen hospitals such as Beers describes, personnel such as he tries to evoke for us—and in so-called progressive, reasonably affluent southern New England; indeed, not many miles from the nation's oldest and most prestigious university.

A particular mind did indeed "find itself"—first by working its way out of the "slough of despond." Beers ascended to mania, then descended to the everyday life of so-called normal people, for whom boredom and a lack of inspiration and energy are an expectable part of fate, and for whom, often enough, dramatic outbursts of emotional feeling must be refused, in favor of a more subdued kind of dissatisfaction—Freud's famous (and inevitable) "discontents" which are, naturally, the price of what gets called "civilization." For Beers, "recovery" did not mean a walk across the street, so to speak—the red-faced, ashamed disavowal of what was. He lived at a time when mental illness was a mark of sin. He had to deal not only with the pain of psychosis, but with the social doubts and censure which had to come his way upon recovery. He makes clear how lucky he was when that time came—the opportunities which befell a Protestant, Yale-educated native American with reasonably good connections. He might have thoroughly cloaked his psychological past; instead, he wrote this book, a public testimony, a sufferer's witness of sorts, and further, spent the rest of his productive life helping establish what became a social and educational movement devoted to "mental hygiene."

Put differently, he went from persuasive chronicler to ardent, entrepreneurial, sophisticated, pragmatic organizer and reformer. His life offers a good deal of instruction in the ways that American society works. Beers was a shrewd tactician, a sensitive observer of the wealthy and the powerful. He more than took their measure, though. He knew how to address them, earn their trust, win them over—and with that achieved, obtain their terribly significant and decisive philanthropic support. With it came new laws, a host of editorials and articles in important newspapers or magazines, and more generally, a shift in public opinion, a shift in the way ordinary men and women came to think about mental illness, and really, about themselves. With no critical intent, I think it fair to call the Beers of middle age a superb pamphleteer, propagandist, social and political activist—a man who knew how to negotiate those so-called corridors of power rather well.

The end was sad: a collapse into withdrawal, if not outright despair, prompted, maybe, by the biological ravages of old age. For those who want to take a close look at the entire span of this exceptional and arresting life, I strongly recommend as a companion to this autobiography, the recently issued and first-rate biography of Beers by Norman Dain, *Clifford Beers: Advocate for the Insane,* published by the same press that has given us this volume. Beers' life is part of our country's history; he followed Dorothea Dix, and he preceded the spate of literary self-observers who arrived on the American scene after the second World War—Lucy Freeman's *Fight Against Fears,* for example. He was a good writer; he also gave himself, body and soul, to a cause—and so doing, redeemed himself, while managing to educate the rest of us, and even help a good number of us deal better with our wayward lives.

Robert Coles
1980

A MIND THAT FOUND ITSELF

❧ I ❧

This story is derived from as human a document as ever existed; and, because of its uncommon nature, perhaps no one thing contributes so much to its value as its authenticity. It is an autobiography, and more: in part it is a biography; for, in telling the story of my life, I must relate the history of another self— a self which was dominant from my twenty-fourth to my twenty-sixth year. During that period I was unlike what I had been, or what I have been since. The biographical part of my autobiography might be called the history of a mental civil war, which I fought single-handed on a battlefield that lay within the compass of my skull. An Army of Unreason, composed of the cunning and treacherous thoughts of an unfair foe, attacked my bewildered consciousness with cruel persistency, and would have destroyed me, had not a triumphant Reason finally interposed a superior strategy that saved me from my unnatural self.

I am not telling the story of my life just to write a book. I tell it because it seems my plain duty to do so. A narrow escape from death and a seemingly miraculous return to health after an apparently fatal illness are enough to make a man ask himself: For what purpose was my life spared? That question I have asked myself, and this book is, in part, an answer.

I was born shortly after sunset about thirty years ago. My ancestors, natives of England, settled in this country not long after the *Mayflower* first sailed into Plymouth Harbor. And the blood of these ancestors, by time and the happy union of a Northern man and a Southern woman—my parents—has perforce been blended into blood truly American.

The first years of my life were, in most ways, not unlike those of other American boys, except as a tendency to worry made them so. Though the fact is now difficult for me to believe, I was painfully shy. When first I put on short trousers, I felt that the eyes of the world were on me; and to escape them I hid behind convenient pieces of furniture while in the house and, so I am told, even sidled close to fences when I walked along the street. With my shyness there was a degree of self-consciousness which put me at a disadvantage in any family or social gathering. I talked little and was ill at ease when others spoke to me.

Like many other sensitive and somewhat introspective children, I passed through a brief period of morbid righteousness. In a game of "one-old-cat," the side on which I played was defeated. On a piece of scantling which lay in the lot where the contest took place, I scratched the score. Afterwards it occurred to me that my inscription was perhaps misleading and would make my side appear to be the winner. I went back and corrected the ambiguity. On finding in an old tool chest at home a coin or medal on which there appeared the text, "Put away the works of darkness and put on the armour of light," my sense of religious propriety was offended. It seemed a sacrilege to use in this way such a high sentiment, so I destroyed the coin.

I early took upon myself, mentally at least, many of the cares and worries of those about me. Whether in this I was different from other youngsters who develop a ludicrous, though pathetic, sense of responsibility for the universe, I do not know. But in my case the most extreme instance occurred during a business depression, when the family resources were endangered. I began to fear that my father (than whom a more hopeful man never lived) might commit suicide.

After all, I am not sure that the other side of my nature— the natural, healthy, boyish side—did not develop equally with these timid and morbid tendencies, which are not so very uncommon in childhood. Certainly the natural, boyish side was more in evidence on the surface. I was as good a sport as any of my playfellows in such games as appealed to me, and I went a-fishing when the chance offered. None of my associates thought of me as being shy or morose. But this was because I masked my troubles, though quite unconsciously, under a camouflage of sarcasm and sallies of wit, or, at least what seemed to pass for wit among my immature acquaintances. With grownups, I was at times inclined to be pert, my degree of impudence depending no doubt upon how ill at ease I was and how perfectly at ease I wished to appear. Because of this constant need for appearing happier than I really was, I developed a knack for saying things in an amusing, sometimes an epigrammatic, way. I recall one remark made long before I could possibly have heard of Malthus or have understood his theory regarding birth rate and food supply. Ours being a large family of limited means and, among the five boys of the family, unlimited appetites, we often used the cheaper, though equally nutritious, cuts of meat. On one occasion when the steak was tougher than usual, I epitomized the Malthusian theory by remarking: "I believe in fewer children and better beefsteak!"

One more incident of my boyhood days may assist the reader to make my acquaintance. In my early teens I was, for one year, a member of a boy choir. Barring my voice, I was a good chorister, and, like all good choirboys, I was distinguished by that seraphic passiveness from which a reaction of some kind is to be expected immediately after a service or rehearsal. On one occasion this reaction in me manifested itself in a fist fight with a fellow choir-boy. Though I cannot recall the time when I have not relished verbal encounters, physical encounters had never been to my taste, and I did not seek this fight. My assailant really goaded me into it. If the honors were not mine, at least I must have acquitted myself creditably, for an interested passer-by made a remark which I have never forgotten. "That boy is all right after he gets started," he said. About twelve years later I did get started, and could that passer-by have seen me on any one of several occasions, he would have had the satisfaction of knowing that his was a prophetic eye.

At the usual age, I entered a public grammar school in New Haven, Connecticut, where I graduated in 1891. In the fall of that year I entered the High School of the same city. My school courses were completed with as little trouble as scholastic distinction. I always managed to gain promotion, however, when it was due; and, though few of my teachers credited me with real ability, they were always able to detect a certain latent capacity, which they evidently believed would one day develop sufficiently to prevent me from disgracing them.

Upon entering the High School I had such ambitions as any schoolboy is apt to have. I wished to secure an election to a given secret society; that gained, I wished to become business manager of a monthly magazine published by that society. In these ambitions I succeeded. For one of my age I had more than an average love of business. Indeed, I deliberately set about learning to play the guitar well enough to become eligible for membership in the Banjo Club—and this for no more aesthetic purpose than to place myself in line for the position of manager, to which I was later elected.

In athletics there was but one game, tennis, in which I was actively interested. Its quick give-and-take suited my temperament, and so fond was I of it that during one summer I played not fewer than four thousand games. As I had an aptitude for tennis and devoted more time to it than did any of my school-mates, it was not surprising that I acquired skill enough to win the school championship during my senior year. But that success was not due entirely to my superiority as a player. It was due in part to what I considered unfair treatment; and the fact well illustrates a certain trait of character which has often stood me in good stead. Among the spectators at the final match of the tournament were several girls. These schoolmates, who lived in my neighborhood, had mistaken for snobbishness a certain boyish diffidence for which few people gave me credit. When we passed each other, almost daily, this group of girls and I, our mutual sign of recognition was a look in an opposite direction. Now my opponent was well liked by these same girls and was entitled to their support. Accordingly they applauded his good plays, which was fair. They did not applaud my good plays, which was also fair. But what was not fair was that they should applaud my bad plays. Their doing so roiled my blood, and thanks to those who would have had me lose, I won.

In June, 1894, I received a high school diploma. Shortly afterwards I took my examination for Yale, and the following September entered the Sheffield Scientific School, in a non-technical course.

The last week of June, 1894, was an important one in my life. An event then occurred which undoubtedly changed my career completely. It was the direct cause of my mental collapse six years later, and of the distressing and, in some instances, strange and delightful experiences on which this book is based. The event was the illness of an older brother, who, late in June, 1894, was stricken with what was thought to be epilepsy. Few diseases can so disorganize a household and distress its members. My brother had enjoyed perfect health up to the time he was stricken; and, as there had never been a suggestion of epilepsy, or any like disease, in either branch of the family, the affliction came as a bolt from a clear sky. Everything possible was done to effect a cure, but without avail. On July 4th, 1900, he died, after a six years' illness, two years of which were spent at home, one year in a trip around the world in a sailing vessel, and most of the remainder on a farm near Hartford. The doctors finally decided that a tumor at the base of the brain had caused his malady and his death.

As I was in college when my brother was first stricken, I had more time at my disposal than the other members of the family, and for that reason spent much of it with him. Though his attacks during the first year occurred only at night, the fear that they might occur during the day, in public, affected my nerves from the beginning.

Now, if a brother who had enjoyed perfect health all his life could be stricken with epilepsy, what was to prevent my being similarly afflicted? This was the thought that soon got possession of my mind. The more I considered it, the more nervous I became; and the more nervous, the more convinced that my own breakdown was only a matter of time. Doomed to what I then considered a living death, I thought of epilepsy, I dreamed epilepsy, until thousands of times during the six years that this disquieting idea persisted, my overwrought imagination seemed to drag me to the very verge of an attack. Yet at no time during my life have these early fears been realized.

For the fourteen months succeeding the time my brother was first stricken, I was greatly harassed with fear; but not until later did my nerves really conquer me. I remember distinctly when the break came. It happened in November, 1895, during a recitation in German. That hour in the class room was one of the most disagreeable I ever experienced. It seemed as if my nerves had snapped, like so many minute bands of rubber stretched beyond their elastic limit. Had I had the courage to leave the room, I should have done so; but I sat as if paralyzed until the class was dismissed.

That term I did not again attend recitations. Continuing my studies at home, I passed satisfactory examinations, which enabled me to resume my place in the class room the following January. During the remainder of my college years I seldom entered a recitation room with any other feeling than that of dread, though the absolute assurance that I should not be called upon to recite did somewhat relieve my anxiety in some classes. The professors, whom I had told about my state of health and the cause of it, invariably treated me with consideration; but, though I believe they never doubted the genuineness of my excuse, it was no easy matter to keep them convinced for almost two-thirds of my college course. My inability to recite was not due usually to any lack of preparation. However well prepared I might be, the moment I was called upon, a mingling of a thousand disconcerting sensations, and the distinct thought that at last the dread attack was at hand, would suddenly intervene and deprive me of all but the power to say, "Not prepared." Weeks would pass without any other record being placed opposite my name than a zero, or a blank indicating that I had not been called upon at all. Occasionally, however, a professor, in justice to himself and to the other students, would insist that I recite, and at such times I managed to make enough of a recitation to hold my place in the class.

When I entered Yale, I had four definite ambitions: first, to secure an election to a coveted secret society; second, to become one of the editors of the *Yale Record,* an illustrated humorous bi-weekly; third (granting that I should succeed in this latter ambition), to convince my associates that I should have the position of business manager—an office which I sought, not for the honor, but because I believed it would enable me to earn an amount of money at least equal to the cost of tuition for my years at Yale; fourth (and this was my chief ambition), to win my diploma within the prescribed time. These four ambitions I fortunately achieved.

A man's college days, collectively, are usually his happiest. Most of mine were not happy. Yet I look back upon them with great satisfaction, for I feel that I was fortunate enough to absorb some of that intangible, but very real, element known as the "Yale spirit." This has helped to keep Hope alive within me during my most discouraged moments, and has ever since made the accomplishment of my purpose seem easy and sure.

~II~

On the thirtieth day of June, 1897, I graduated at Yale. Had I then realized that I was a sick man, I could and would have taken a rest. But, in a way, I had become accustomed to the ups and downs of a nervous existence, and, as I could not really afford a rest, six days after my graduation I entered upon the duties of a clerk in the office of the Collector of Taxes in the city of New Haven. I was fortunate in securing such a position at that time, for the hours were comparatively short and the work as congenial as any could have been under the circumstances. I entered the Tax Office with the intention of staying only until such time as I might secure a position in New York. About a year later I secured the desired position. After remaining in it for eight months I left it, in order to take a position which seemed to offer a field of endeavor more to my taste. From May, 1899, till the middle of June, 1900, I was a clerk in one of the smaller life-insurance companies, whose home office was within a stone's throw of what some men consider the center of the universe. To be in the very heart of the financial district of New York appealed strongly to my imagination. As a result of the contagious ideals of Wall Street, the making of money was then a passion with me. I wished to taste the bittersweet of power based on wealth.

For the first eighteen months of my life in New York, my health seemed no worse than it had been during the preceding three years. But the old dread still possessed me. I continued to have my more and less nervous days, weeks, and months. In March, 1900, however, there came a change for the worse. At that time I had a severe attack of grippe which incapacitated me for two weeks. As was to be expected in my case, this illness seriously depleted my vitality, and left me in a frightfully depressed condition—a depression which continued to grow upon me until the final crash came, on June 23rd, 1900. The events of that day, seemingly disastrous as then viewed, but evidently all for the best as the issue proved, forced me along paths traveled by thousands, but comprehended by few.

I had continued to perform my clerical duties until June 15th. On that day I was compelled to stop, and that at once. I had reached a point where my will had to capitulate to Unreason— that unscrupulous usurper. My previous five years as a neurasthenic had led me to believe that I had experienced all the disagreeable sensations an overworked and unstrung nervous system could suffer. But on this day several new and terrifying sensations seized me and rendered me all but helpless. My condition, however, was not apparent even to those who worked with me at the same desk. I remember trying to speak and at times finding myself unable to give utterance to my thoughts. Though I was able to answer questions, that fact hardly diminished my feeling of apprehension, for a single failure in an attempt to speak will stagger any man, no matter what his state of health. I tried to copy certain records in the day's work, but my hand was too unsteady, and I found it difficult to read the words and figures presented to my tired vision in blurred confusion.

That afternoon, conscious that some terrible calamity was impending, but not knowing what would be its nature, I performed a very curious act. Certain early literary efforts which had failed of publication in the college paper, but which I had jealously cherished for several years, I utterly destroyed. Then, after a hurried arrangement of my affairs, I took an early afternoon train, and was soon in New Haven. Home life did not make me better, and, except for three or four short walks, I did not go out of the house at all until June 23d, when I went in a most unusual way. To relatives I said little about my state of health, beyond the general statement that I had never felt worse —a statement which, when made by a neurasthenic, means much, but proves little. For five years I had had my ups and downs, and both my relatives and myself had begun to look upon these as things which would probably be corrected in and by time.

The day after my home-coming I made up my mind, or that part of it which was still within my control, that the time had come to quit business entirely and take a rest of months. I even arranged with a younger brother to set out at once for some quiet place in the White Mountains, where I hoped to steady my shattered nerves. At this time I felt as though in a tremor from head to foot, and the thought that I was about to have an epileptic attack constantly recurred. On more than one occasion I said to friends that I would rather die than live an epileptic; yet, if I rightly remember, I never declared the actual fear that I was doomed to bear such an affliction. Though I held the mad belief that I should suffer epilepsy, I held the sane hope, amounting to belief, that I should escape it. This fact may account, in a measure, for my six years of endurance.

On the 18th of June I felt so much worse that I went to my bed and stayed there until the 23d. During the night of the 18th my persistent dread became a false belief—a delusion. What I had long expected I now became convinced had at last occurred. I believed myself to be a confirmed epileptic, and that conviction was stronger than any ever held by a sound intellect. The half-resolve, made before my mind was actually impaired, namely, that I would kill myself rather than live the life I dreaded, now divided my attention with the belief that the stroke had fallen. From that time my one thought was to hasten the end, for I felt that I should lose the chance to die should relatives find me in an attack of epilepsy.

Considering the state of my mind and my inability at that time to appreciate the enormity of such an end as I half contemplated, my suicidal purpose was not entirely selfish. That I had never seriously contemplated suicide is proved by the fact that I had not provided myself with the means of accomplishing it, despite my habit, which has long been remarked by my friends, of preparing even for unlikely contingencies. So far as I had the control of my faculties, it must be admitted that I deliberated; but, strictly speaking, the rash act which followed cannot correctly be called an attempt at suicide—for how can a man who is not himself kill himself?

Soon my disordered brain was busy with schemes for death. I distinctly remember one which included a row on Lake Whitney, near New Haven. This I intended to take in the most unstable boat obtainable. Such a craft could be easily upset, and I should so bequeath to relatives and friends a sufficient number of reasonable doubts to rob my death of the usual stigma. I also remember searching for some deadly drug which I hoped to find about the house. But the quantity and quality of what I found were not such as I dared to trust. I then thought of severing my jugular vein, even going so far as to test against my throat the edge of a razor which, after the deadly impulse first asserted itself, I had secreted in a convenient place. I really wished to die, but so uncertain and ghastly a method did not appeal to me. Nevertheless, had I felt sure that in my tremulous frenzy I could accomplish the act with skillful dispatch, I should at once have ended my troubles.

My imaginary attacks were now recurring with distracting frequency, and I was in constant fear of discovery. During these three or four days I slept scarcely at all—even the medicine given to induce sleep having little effect. Though inwardly frenzied, I gave no outward sign of my condition. Most of the time I remained quietly in bed. I spoke but seldom. I had practically, though not entirely, lost the power of speech; but my almost unbroken silence aroused no suspicions as to the seriousness of my condition.

By a process of elimination, all suicidal methods but one had at last been put aside. On that one my mind now centered. My room was on the fourth floor of the house—one of a block of five—in which my parents lived. The house stood several feet back from the street. The sills of my windows were a little more than thirty feet above the ground. Under one was a flag pavement, extending from the house to the front gate. Under the other was a rectangular coal-hole covered with an iron grating. This was surrounded by flagging over a foot in width; and connecting it and the pavement proper was another flag. So that all along the front of the house, stone or iron filled a space at no point less than two feet in width. It required little calculation to determine how slight the chance of surviving a fall from either of those two windows.

About dawn I arose. Stealthily I approached a window, pushed open the blinds, and looked out—and down. Then I closed the blinds as noiselessly as possible and crept back to bed: I had not yet become so irresponsible that I dared to take the leap. Scarcely had I pulled up the covering when a watchful relative entered my room, drawn thither perhaps by that protecting prescience which love inspires. I thought her words revealed a suspicion that she had heard me at the window, but speechless as I was I had enough speech to deceive her. For of what account are Truth and Love when Life itself has ceased to seem desirable?

The dawn soon hid itself in the brilliancy of a perfect June day. Never had I seen a brighter—to look at; never a darker—to live through—or a better to die upon. Its very perfection and the songs of the robins, which at that season were plentiful in the neighborhood, served but to increase my despair and make me the more willing to die. As the day wore on, my anguish became more intense, but I managed to mislead those about me by uttering a word now and then, and feigning to read a newspaper, which to me, however, appeared an unintelligible jumble of type. My brain was in a ferment. It felt as if pricked by a million needles at white heat. My whole body felt as though it would be torn apart by the terrific nervous strain under which I labored.

Shortly after noon, dinner having been served, my mother entered the room and asked me if she should bring me some dessert. I assented. It was not that I cared for the dessert; I had no appetite. I wished to get her out of the room, for I believed myself to be on the verge of another attack. She left at once. I knew that in two or three minutes she would return. The crisis seemed at hand. It was now or never for liberation. She had probably descended one of three flights of stairs when, with the mad desire to dash my brains out on the pavement below, I rushed to that window which was directly over the flag walk. Providence must have guided my movements, for in some otherwise unaccountable way, on the very point of hurling myself out bodily, I chose to drop feet foremost instead. With my fingers I clung for a moment to the sill. Then I let go. In falling my body turned so as to bring my right side toward the building. I struck the ground a little more than two feet from the foundation of the house, and at least three to the left of the point from which I started. Missing the stone pavement by not more than three or four inches, I struck on comparatively soft earth. My position must have been almost upright, for both heels struck the ground squarely. The concussion slightly crushed one heel bone and broke most of the small bones in the arch of each foot, but there was no mutilation of the flesh. As my feet struck the ground my right hand struck hard against the front of the house, and it is probable that these three points of contact, dividing the force of the shock, prevented my back from being broken. As it was, it narrowly escaped a fracture and, for several weeks afterward, it felt as if powdered glass had been substituted for cartilage between the vertebræ.

I did not lose consciousness even for a second, and the demoniacal dread, which had possessed me from June, 1894, until this fall to earth just six years later, was dispelled the instant I struck the ground. At no time since have I experienced one of my imaginary attacks; nor has my mind even for a moment entertained such an idea. The little demon which had tortured me relentlessly for so many years evidently lacked the stamina which I must have had to survive the shock of my suddenly arrested flight through space. That the very delusion which drove me to a death-loving desperation should so suddenly vanish would seem to indicate that many a suicide might be averted if the person contemplating it could find the proper assistance when such a crisis impends.

ᘖ III ᘗ

It was squarely in front of the dining-room window that I fell, and those at dinner were, of course, startled. It took them a second or two to realize what had happened. Then my younger brother rushed out, and with others carried me into the house. Naturally that dinner was permanently interrupted. A mattress was placed on the floor of the dining room and I on that, suffering intensely. I said little, but what I said was significant. "I thought I had epilepsy!" was my first remark; and several times I said, "I wish it was over!" For I believed that my death was only a question of hours. To the doctors, who soon arrived, I said, "My back is broken!"—raising myself slightly, however, as I said so.

An ambulance was summoned and I was placed in it. Because of the nature of my injuries it had to proceed slowly. The trip of a mile and a half seemed interminable, but finally I arrived at Grace Hospital and was placed in a room which soon became a chamber of torture. It was on the second floor; and the first object to engage my attention and stir my imagination was a man who appeared outside my window and placed in position several heavy iron bars. These were, it seems, thought necessary for my protection, but at that time no such idea occurred to me. My mind was in a delusional state, ready and eager to seize upon any external stimulus as a pretext for its

16

wild inventions, and that barred window started a terrible strain of delusions which persisted for seven hundred and ninety-eight days. During that period my mind imprisoned both mind and body in a dungeon than which none was ever more secure.

Knowing that those who attempt suicide are usually placed under arrest, I believed myself under legal restraint. I imagined that at any moment I might be taken to court to face some charge lodged against me by the local police. Every act of those about me seemed to be a part of what, in police parlance, is commonly called the "Third Degree." The hot poultices placed upon my feet and ankles threw me into a profuse perspiration, and my very active association of mad ideas convinced me that I was being "sweated"—another police term which I had often seen in the newspapers. I inferred that this third-degree sweating process was being inflicted in order to extort some kind of a confession, though what my captors wished me to confess I could not for my life imagine. As I was really in a state of delirium, with high fever, I had an insatiable thirst. The only liquids given me were hot saline solutions. Though there was good reason for administering these, I believed they were designed for no other purpose than to increase my sufferings, as part of the same inquisitorial process. But had a confession been due, I could hardly have made it, for that part of my brain which controls the power of speech was seriously affected, and was soon to be further disabled by my ungovernable thoughts. Only an occasional word did I utter.

Certain hallucinations of hearing, or "false voices," added to my torture. Within my range of hearing, but beyond the reach of my understanding, there was a hellish vocal hum. Now and then I would recognize the subdued voice of a friend; now and then I would hear the voices of some I believed were not friends. All these referred to me and uttered what I could not clearly distinguish, but knew must be imprecations. Ghostly rappings on the walls and ceiling of my room punctuated unintelligible mumblings of invisible persecutors.

I remember distinctly my delusion of the following day— Sunday. I seemed to be no longer in the hospital. In some mysterious way I had been spirited aboard a huge ocean liner. I first discovered this when the ship was in mid-ocean. The day was clear, the sea apparently calm, but for all that the ship was slowly sinking. And it was I, of course, who had created the situation which must turn out fatally for all, unless the coast of Europe could be reached before the water in the hold should extinguish the fires. How had this peril overtaken us? Simply enough: During the night I had in some way—a way still unknown to me—opened a porthole below the water-line; and those in charge of the vessel seemed powerless to close it. Every now and then I could hear parts of the ship give way under the strain. I could hear the air hiss and whistle spitefully under the resistless impact of the invading waters; I could hear the crashing of timbers as partitions were wrecked; and as the water rushed in at one place I could see, at another, scores of helpless passengers swept overboard into the sea—my unintended victims. I believed that I, too, might at any moment be swept away. That I was not thrown into the sea by vengeful fellow-passengers was, I thought, due to their desire to keep me alive until, if possible, land should be reached, when a more painful death could be inflicted upon me.

While aboard my phantom ship I managed in some way to establish an electric railway system; and the trolley cars which passed the hospital were soon running along the deck of my ocean liner, carrying passengers from the places of peril to what seemed places of comparative safety at the bow. Every time I heard a car pass the hospital, one of mine went clanging along the ship's deck.

My feverish imaginings were no less remarkable than the external stimuli which excited them. As I have since ascertained, there were just outside my room an elevator and near it a speaking-tube. Whenever the speaking-tube was used from another part of the building, the summoning whistle conveyed to my mind the idea of the exhaustion of air in a ship-compartment, and the opening and shutting of the elevator door completed the illusion of a ship fast going to pieces. But the ship my mind was on never reached any shore, nor did she sink. Like a mirage she vanished, and again I found myself safe in my bed at the hospital. "Safe," did I say? Scarcely that—for deliverance from one impending disaster simply meant immediate precipitation into another.

My delirium gradually subsided, and four or five days after the 23d the doctors were able to set my broken bones. The operation suggested new delusions. Shortly before the adjustment of the plaster casts, my legs, for obvious reasons, were shaved from shin to calf. This unusual tonsorial operation I read for a sign of degradation—associating it with what I had heard of the treatment of murderers and with similar customs in barbarous countries. It was about this time also that strips of court-plaster, in the form of a cross, were placed on my forehead, which had been slightly scratched in my fall, and this, of course, I interpreted as a brand of infamy.

Had my health been good, I should at this time have been participating in the Triennial of my class at Yale. Indeed, I was a member of the Triennial Committee and though, when I left New York on June 15th, I had been feeling terribly ill, I had then hoped to take part in the celebration. The class reunions were held on Tuesday, June 26th—three days after my collapse. Those familiar with Yale customs know that the Harvard baseball game is one of the chief events of the commencement season. Headed by brass bands, all the classes whose reunions fall in the same year march to the Yale Athletic Field to see the game and renew their youth—using up as much vigor in one delirious day as would insure a ripe old age if less prodigally expended. These classes, with their bands and cheering, accompanied by thousands of other vociferating enthusiasts, march through West Chapel Street—the most direct route from the Campus to the Field. It is upon this line of march that Grace Hospital is situated, and I knew that on the day of the game the Yale thousands would pass the scene of my incarceration.

I have endured so many days of the most exquisite torture that I hesitate to distinguish among them by degrees; each deserves its own unique place, even as a Saint's Day in the calendar of an olden Spanish inquisitor. But, if the palm is to be awarded to any, June 26th, 1900, perhaps has the first claim.

My state of mind at that time might be pictured thus: The criminal charge of attempted suicide stood against me on June 23rd. By the 26th many other and worse charges had accumulated. The public believed me the most despicable member of my race. The papers were filled with accounts of my misdeeds. The thousands of collegians gathered in the city, many of whom I knew personally, loathed the very thought that a Yale man should so disgrace his Alma Mater. And when they approached the hospital on their way to the Athletic Field, I concluded that it was their intention to take me from my bed, drag me to the lawn, and there tear me limb from limb. Few incidents during my unhappiest years are more vividly or circumstantially impressed upon my memory. The fear, to be sure, was absurd, but in the lurid lexicon of Unreason there is no such word as "absurd." Believing, as I did, that I had dishonored Yale and forfeited the privilege of being numbered among her sons, it was not surprising that the college cheers which filled the air that afternoon, and in which only a few days earlier I had hoped to join, struck terror to my heart.

Naturally I was suspicious of all about me, and became more so each day. But not until about a month later did I refuse to recognize my relatives. While I was at Grace Hospital, my father and eldest brother called almost every day to see me, and, though I said little, I still accepted them in their proper characters. I remember well a conversation one morning with my father. The words I uttered were few, but full of meaning. Shortly before this time my death had been momentarily expected. I still believed that I was surely about to die as a result of my injuries, and I wished in some way to let my father know that, despite my apparently ignominious end, I appreciated all that he had done for me during my life. Few men, I believe, ever had a more painful time in expressing their feelings than I had on that occasion. I had but little control over my mind, and my power of speech was impaired. My father sat beside my bed. Looking up at him, I said, "You have been a good father to me."

"I have always tried to be," was his characteristic reply.

After the broken bones had been set, and the first effects of the severe shock I had sustained had worn off, I began to gain strength. About the third week I was able to sit up and was occasionally taken out of doors. But each day, and especially during the hours of the night, my delusions increased in force and variety. The world was fast becoming to me a stage on which every human being within the range of my senses seemed to be playing a part, and that a part which would lead not only to my destruction (for which I cared little), but also to the ruin of all with whom I had ever come in contact. In the month of July several thunder storms occurred. To me the thunder was "stage" thunder, the lightning man-made, and the accompanying rain due to some clever contrivance of my persecutors. There was a chapel connected with the hospital—or at least a room where religious services were held every Sunday. To me the hymns were funeral dirges; and the mumbled prayers, faintly audible, were in behalf of every sufferer in the world but one.

It was my eldest brother who looked after my care and interests during my entire illness. Toward the end of July, he informed me that I was to be taken home again. I must have given him an incredulous look, for he said, "Don't you think we can take you home? Well, we can and will." Believing myself in the hands of the police, I did not see how that was possible. Nor did I have any desire to return. That a man who had disgraced his family should again enter his old home and expect his relatives to treat him as though nothing were changed, was a thought against which my soul rebelled; and, when the day came for my return, I fought my brother and the doctor feebly as they lifted me from the bed. But I soon submitted, was placed in a carriage, and driven to the house I had left a month earlier.

For a few hours my mind was calmer than it had been. But my new-found ease was soon dispelled by the appearance of a nurse—one of several who had attended me at the hospital. Though at home and surrounded by relatives, I jumped to the conclusion that I was still under police surveillance. At my request my brother had promised not to engage any nurse who had been in attendance at the hospital. The difficulty of procuring any other led him to disregard my request, which at the time he held simply as a whim. But he did not disregard it entirely, for the nurse selected had merely acted as a substitute on one occasion, and then only for about an hour. That was long enough, though, for my memory to record her image.

Finding myself still under surveillance, I soon jumped to a second conclusion, namely, that this was no brother of mine at all. He instantly appeared in the light of a sinister double, acting as a detective. After that I refused absolutely to speak to him again, and this repudiation I extended to all other relatives, friends and acquaintances. If the man I had accepted as my brother was spurious, so was everybody—that was my deduction. For more than two years I was without relatives or friends, in fact, without a world, except that one created by my own mind from the chaos that reigned within it.

While I was at Grace Hospital, it was my sense of hearing which was most disturbed. But soon after I was placed in my room at home, *all* of my senses became perverted. I still heard the "false voices"—which were doubly false, for Truth no longer existed. The tricks played upon me by my senses of taste, touch, smell, and sight were the source of great mental anguish. None of my food had its usual flavor. This soon led to that common delusion that some of it contained poison—not deadly poison, for I knew that my enemies hated me too much to allow me the boon of death, but poison sufficient to aggravate my discomfort. At breakfast I had cantaloupe, liberally sprinkled with salt. The salt seemed to pucker my mouth, and I believed it to be powdered alum. Usually, with my supper, sliced peaches were served. Though there was sugar on the peaches, salt would have done as well. Salt, sugar, and powdered alum had become the same to me.

Familiar materials had acquired a different "feel." In the dark, the bed sheets at times seemed like silk. As I had not been born with a golden spoon in my mouth, or other accessories of a useless luxury, I believed the detectives had provided these silken sheets for some hostile purpose of their own. What that purpose was I could not divine, and my very inability to arrive at a satisfactory conclusion stimulated my brain to the assembling of disturbing thoughts in an almost endless train.

Imaginary breezes struck my face, gentle, but not welcome, most of them from parts of the room where currents of air could not possibly originate. They seemed to come from cracks in the walls and ceiling and annoyed me exceedingly. I thought them in some way related to that ancient method of torture by which water is allowed to strike the victim's forehead, a drop at a time, until death releases him. For a while my sense of smell added to my troubles. The odor of burning human flesh and other pestilential fumes seemed to assail me.

My sense of sight was subjected to many weird and uncanny effects. Phantasmagoric visions made their visitations throughout the night, for a time with such regularity that I used to await their coming with a certain restrained curiosity. I was not entirely unaware that something was ailing with my mind. Yet these illusions of sight I took for the work of detectives, who sat up nights racking their brains in order to rack and utterly wreck my own with a cruel and unfair Third Degree.

Handwriting on the wall has ever struck terror to the hearts of even sane men. I remember as one of my most unpleasant experiences that I began to see handwriting on the sheets of my bed staring me in the face, and not me alone, but also the spurious relatives who often stood or sat near me. On each fresh sheet placed over me I would soon begin to see words, sentences, and signatures, all in my own handwriting. Yet I could not decipher any of the words, and this fact dismayed me, for I firmly believed that those who stood about could read them all and found them to be incriminating evidence.

I imagined that these visionlike effects, with few exceptions, were produced by a magic lantern controlled by some of my myriad persecutors. The lantern was rather a cinematographic contrivance. Moving pictures, often brilliantly colored, were thrown on the ceiling of my room and sometimes on the sheets of my bed. Human bodies, dismembered and gory, were one of the most common of these. All this may have been due to the fact that, as a boy, I had fed my imagination on the sensational news of the day as presented in the public press. Despite the heavy penalty which I now paid for thus loading my mind, I believe this unwise indulgence gave a breadth and variety to my peculiar psychological experience which it otherwise would have lacked. For with an insane ingenuity I managed to connect myself with almost every crime of importance of which I had ever read.

Dismembered human bodies were not alone my bedfellows at this time. I remember one vision of vivid beauty. Swarms of butterflies and large and gorgeous moths appeared on the sheets. I wished that the usually unkind operator would continue to show these pretty creatures. Another pleasing vision appeared about twilight several days in succession. I can trace it directly to impressions gained in early childhood. The quaint pictures by Kate Greenaway—little children in attractive dress, playing in old-fashioned gardens—would float through space just outside my windows. The pictures were always accompanied by the gleeful shouts of real children in the neighborhood, who, before being sent to bed by watchful parents, devoted the last hour of the day to play. It doubtless was their shouts that stirred my memories of childhood and brought forth these pictures.

In my chamber of intermittent horrors and momentary delights, uncanny occurrences were frequent. I believed there was some one who at fall of night secreted himself under my bed. That in itself was not peculiar, as sane persons at one time or another are troubled by that same notion. But *my* bed-fellow—

under the bed—was a detective; and he spent most of the time during the night pressing pieces of ice against my injured heels, to precipitate, as I thought, my overdue confession.

The piece of ice in the pitcher of water which usually stood on the table sometimes clinked against the pitcher's side as its center of gravity shifted through melting. It was many days before I reasoned out the cause of this sound; and until I did I supposed it was produced by some mechanical device resorted to by the detectives for a purpose. Thus the most trifling occurrence assumed for me vast significance.

❦ V ❧

After remaining at home for about a month, during which time I showed no improvement mentally, though I did gain physically, I was taken to a private sanatorium. My destination was frankly disclosed to me. But my habit of disbelief had now become fixed, and I thought myself on the way to a trial in New York City, for some one of the many crimes with which I stood charged.

My emotions on leaving New Haven were, I imagine, much the same as those of a condemned but penitent criminal who looks upon the world for the last time. The day was hot, and, as we drove to the railway station, the blinds on most of the houses in the streets through which we passed were seen to be closed. The reason for this was not then apparent to me. I thought I saw an unbroken line of deserted houses, and I imagined that their desertion had been deliberately planned as a sign of displeasure on the part of their former occupants. As citizens of New Haven, I supposed them bitterly ashamed of such a despicable townsman as myself. Because of the early hour, the streets were practically deserted. This fact, too, I interpreted to my own disadvantage. As the carriage crossed the main business thoroughfare, I took what I believed to be my last look at that part of my native city.

From the carriage I was carried to the train and placed in the smoking car in the last seat on the right-hand side. The back of the seat next in front was reversed so that my legs might be placed in a comfortable position, and one of the boards used by card-playing travelers was placed beneath them as a support. With a consistent degree of suspicion I paid particular attention to a blue mark on the face of the railroad ticket held by my custodian. I took it to be a means of identification for use in court.

That one's memory may perform its function in the grip of Unreason itself is proved by the fact that my memory retains an impression, and an accurate one, of virtually everything that befell me, except when under the influence of an anæsthetic or in the unconscious hours of undisturbed sleep. Important events, trifling conversations, and more trifling thoughts of my own are now recalled with ease and accuracy; whereas, prior to my illness and until a strange experience to be recorded later, mine was an ordinary memory when it was not noticeably poor. At school and in college I stood lowest in those studies in which success depended largely upon this faculty. Psychiatrists inform me that it is not unusual for those suffering as I did to retain accurate impressions of their experiences while ill. To laymen this may seem almost miraculous, yet it is not so; nor is it even remarkable. Assuming that an insane person's memory is capable of recording impressions at all, remembrance for one in the torturing grip of delusions of persecution should be doubly easy. This deduction is in accord with the accepted psychological law that the retention of an impression in the memory depends largely upon the intensity of the impression itself, and the frequency of its repetition. Fear to speak, lest I should incriminate myself and others, gave to my impressions the requisite intensity, and the daily recurrence of the same general line of thought served to fix all impressions in my then supersensitive memory.

Shortly before seven in the morning, on the way to the sanatorium, the train passed through a manufacturing center. Many workmen were lounging in front of a factory, most of them reading newspapers. I believed these papers contained an account of me and my crimes, and I thought everyone along the route knew who I was and what I was, and that I was on that train. Few seemed to pay any attention to me, yet this very fact looked to be a part of some well-laid plan of the detectives.

The sanatorium to which I was going was in the country. When a certain station was reached, I was carried from the train to a carriage. At that moment I caught sight of a former college acquaintance, whose appearance I thought was designed to let me know that Yale, which I believed I had disgraced, was one of the powers behind my throne of torture.

Soon after I reached my room in the sanatorium, the supervisor entered. Drawing a table close to the bed, he placed on it a slip of paper which he asked me to sign. I looked upon this as a trick of the detectives to get a specimen of my handwriting. I now know that the signing of the slip is a legal requirement, with which every patient is supposed to comply upon entering such an institution—private in character—unless be has been committed by some court. The exact wording of this "voluntary commitment" I do not now recall; but, it was, in substance, an agreement to abide by the rules of the institution—whatever *they* were—and to submit to such restraint as might be deemed necessary. Had I not felt the weight of the world on my shoulders, I believe my sense of humor would have caused me to laugh outright; for the signing of such an agreement by one so situated was, even to my mind, a farce. After much coaxing I was induced to go so far as to take the pen in my hand. There I again hesitated. The supervisor apparently thought I might write with more ease if the paper were placed on a book. And so I might, had he selected a book of a different title. One more likely to arouse suspicions in my mind could not have been found in a search of the Congressional Library. I had left New York on June 15th, and it was in the direction of that city that my present trip had taken me. I considered this but the first step of my return under the auspices of its Police Department. "Called Back" was the title of the book that stared me in the face. After refusing for a long time I finally weakened and signed the slip; but I did not place it on the book. To have done that would, in my mind, have been tantamount to giving consent to extradition; and I was in no mood to assist the detectives in their mean work. At what cost had I signed that commitment slip? To me it was the act of signing my own death-warrant.

During the entire time that my delusions of persecution, as they are called, persisted, I could not but respect the mind that had laid out so comprehensive and devilishly ingenious and, at times, artistic a Third Degree as I was called upon to bear. And an innate modesty (more or less fugitive since these peculiar experiences) does not forbid my mentioning the fact that I still respect that mind.

Suffering such as I endured during the month of August in my own home continued with gradually diminishing force during the eight months I remained in this sanatorium. Nevertheless my sufferings during the first four of these eight months was intense. All my senses were still perverted. My sense of sight was the first to right itself—nearly enough, at least, to rob the detectives of their moving pictures. But before the last fitful film had run through my mind, I beheld one which I shall now describe. I can trace it directly to an impression made on my memory about two years earlier, before my breakdown.

Shortly after going to New York to live, I had explored the Eden Musée. One of the most gruesome of the spectacles which I had seen in its famed Chamber of Horrors was a representation of a gorilla, holding in its arms the gory body of a woman. It was that impression which now revived in my mind. But by a process strictly in accordance with Darwin's theory, the Eden Musée gorilla had become a man—in appearance not unlike the beast that had inspired my distorted thought. This man held a bloody dagger which he repeatedly plunged into the woman's breast. The apparition did not terrify me at all. In fact I found it interesting, for I looked upon it as a contrivance of the detectives. Its purpose I could not divine, but this fact did not trouble me, as I reasoned that no additional criminal charges could make my situation worse than it already was.

For a month or two, "false voices" continued to annoy me. And if there is a hell conducted on the principles of my temporary hell, gossipers will one day wish they had attended strictly to their own business. This is not a confession. I am no gossiper, though I cannot deny that I have occasionally gossiped—a little. And this was my punishment: persons in an adjoining room seemed to be repeating the very same things which I had said of others on these communicative occasions. I supposed that those whom I had talked about had in some way found me out, and intended now to take their revenge.

My sense of smell, too, became normal; but my sense of taste was slow in recovering. At each meal, poison was still the *pièce de résistance,* and it was not surprising that I sometimes dallied one, two, or three hours over a meal, and often ended by not eating it at all.

There was, however, another reason for my frequent refusal to take food, in my belief that the detectives had resorted to a more subtle method of detection. They now intended by each article of food to suggest a certain idea, and I was expected to recognize the idea thus suggested. Conviction or acquittal depended upon my correct interpretation of their symbols, and my interpretation was to be signified by my eating, or not eating, the several kinds of food placed before me. To have eaten a burnt crust of bread would have been a confession of arson. Why? Simply because the charred crust suggested fire; and, as bread is the staff of life, would it not be an inevitable deduction that life had been destroyed—destroyed by fire—and that I was the destroyer? On one day to eat a given article of food meant confession. The next day, or the next meal, a refusal to eat it meant confession. This complication of logic made it doubly difficult for me to keep from incriminating myself and others.

It can easily be seen that I was between several devils and the deep sea. To eat or not to eat perplexed me more than the problem conveyed by a few shorter words perplexed a certain prince, who, had he lived a few centuries later (out of a book), might have been forced to enter a kingdom where kings and princes are made and unmade on short notice. Indeed, he might have lost his principality entirely—or, at least, his subjects; for, as I later had occasion to observe, the frequency with which a dethroned reason mounts a throne and rules a world is such that self-crowned royalty receives but scant homage from the less elated members of the court.

For several weeks I ate but little. Though the desire for food was not wanting, my mind (that dog-in-the-manger) refused to let me satisfy my hunger. Coaxing by the attendants was of little avail; force was usually of less. But the threat that liquid nourishment would be administered through my nostrils sometimes prevailed, for the attribute of shrewdness was not so utterly lost that I could not choose the less of two evils.

What I looked upon as a gastronomic ruse of the detectives sometimes overcame my fear of eating. Every Sunday ice cream was served with dinner. At the beginning of the meal a large pyramid of it would be placed before me in a saucer several sizes too small. I believed that it was never to be mine unless I first partook of the more substantial fare. As I dallied over the meal, that delicious pyramid would gradually melt, slowly filling the small saucer, which I knew could not long continue to hold all of its original contents. As the melting of the ice cream progressed, I became more indifferent to my eventual fate; and, invariably, before a drop of that precious reward had dripped from the saucer, I had eaten enough of the dinner to prove my title to the seductive dessert. Moreover, during its enjoyment, I no longer cared a whit for charges or convictions of all the crimes in the calendar. This fact is less trifling than it seems; for it proves the value of strategy as opposed to brute and sometimes brutal force, of which I shall presently give some illuminating examples.

☙ VII ❧

Choice of a sanatorium by people of limited means is, unfortunately, very restricted. Though my relatives believed the one in which I was placed was at least fairly well conducted, events proved otherwise. From a modest beginning made not many years previously, it had enjoyed a mushroom growth. About two hundred and fifty patients were harbored in a dozen or more small frame buildings, suggestive of a mill settlement. Outside the limits of a city and in a state where there was lax official supervision, owing in part to faulty laws, the owner of this little settlement of woe had erected a nest of veritable firetraps in which helpless sick people were forced to risk their lives. This was a necessary procedure if the owner was to grind out an exorbitant income on his investment.

The same spirit of economy and commercialism pervaded the entire institution. Its worst manifestation was in the employment of the meanest type of attendant—men willing to work for the paltry wage of eighteen dollars a month. Very seldom did competent attendants consent to work there, and then usually because of a scarcity of profitable employment elsewhere. Providentially for me, such an attendant came upon the scene. This young man, so long as he remained in the good graces of the owner-superintendent, was admittedly one of the best attendants he had ever had. Yet aside from a five-dollar bill which a relative had sent me at Christmas and which I had refused to accept because of my belief that it, like my relatives, was counterfeit—aside from that bill, which was turned over to the attendant by my brother, he received no additional pecuniary rewards. His chief reward lay in his consciousness of the fact that he was protecting me against injustices which surely would have been visited upon me had he quitted his position and left me to the mercies of the owner and his ignorant assistants. Today, with deep appreciation, I contrast the treatment I received at his hands with that which I suffered during the three weeks preceding his appearance on the scene. During that period, no fewer than seven attendants contributed to my misery. Though some of them were perhaps decent enough fellows outside a sickroom, not one had the right to minister to a patient in my condition.

The two who were first put in charge of me did not strike me with their fists or even threaten to do so; but their unconscious lack of consideration for my comfort and peace of mind was torture. They were typical eighteen-dollar-a-month attendants. Another of the same sort, on one occasion, cursed me with a degree of brutality which I prefer not to recall, much less record. And a few days later the climax was appropriately capped when still another attendant perpetrated an outrage which a sane man would have resented to the point of homicide. He was a man of the coarsest type. His hands would have done credit to a longshoreman—fingers knotted and nearly twice the normal size. Because I refused to obey a peremptory command, and this at a time when I habitually refused even on pain of imagined torture to obey or speak, this brute not only cursed me with abandon, he deliberately spat upon me. I was a mental incompetent, but like many others in a similar position I was both by antecedents and by training a gentleman. Vitriol could not have seared my flesh more deeply than the venom of this human viper stung my soul! Yet, as I was rendered speechless by delusions, I could not offer so much as a word of protest.

I trust that it is not now too late, however, to protest in behalf of the thousands of outraged patients in private and state hospitals whose mute submission to such indignities has never been recorded.

Of the readiness of an unscrupulous owner to employ inferior attendants, I shall offer a striking illustration. The capable attendant who acted as my protector at this sanatorium has given me an affidavit embodying certain facts which, of course, I could not have known at the time of their occurrence. The gist of this sworn statement is as follows: One day a man—seemingly a tramp—approached the main building of the sanatorium and inquired for the owner. He soon found him, talked with him a few minutes, and an hour or so later he was sitting at the bedside of an old and infirm man. This aged patient had recently been committed to the institution by relatives who had labored under the common delusion that the payment of a considerable sum of money each week would insure kindly treatment. When this tramp-attendant first appeared, all his visible worldly possessions were contained in a small bundle which he carried under his arm. So filthy were his person and his clothes that he received a compulsory bath and another suit before being assigned to duty. He then began to earn his four dollars and fifty cents a week by sitting several hours a day in the room with the aged man, sick unto death. My informant soon engaged him in conversation. What did he learn? First, that the uncouth stranger had never before so much as crossed the threshold of a hospital. His last job had been as a member of a section-gang on a railroad. From the roadbed of a railway to the bedside of a man about to die was indeed a change which might have taxed the adaptability of a more versatile being. But coarse as he was, this unkempt novice did not abuse his charge—except in so far as his inability to interpret or anticipate wants contributed to the sick man's distress. My own attendant, realizing that the patient was suffering for the want of skilled attention, spent a part of his time in this unhappy room, which was but across the hall from my own. The end soon came.

My attendant, who had had training as a nurse, detected the unmistakable signs of impending death. He forthwith informed the owner of the sanatorium that the patient was in a dying condition, and urged him (a doctor) to go at once to the bedside. The doctor refused to comply with the request on the plea that he was at the time "too busy." When at last he did visit the room, the patient was dead. Then came the supervisor, who took charge of the body. As it was being carried from the room the supervisor, the "handy man" of the owner, said: "There goes the best paying patient the institution had; the doctor" (meaning the owner) "was getting eighty-five dollars a week out of him." Of this sum not more than twenty dollars at most, at the time this happened, could be considered as "cost of maintenance." The remaining sixty-five dollars went into the pocket of the owner. Had the man lived for one year, the owner might have pocketed (so far as this one case was concerned) the neat but wicked profit of thirty-three hundred and eighty dollars. And what would the patient have received? The same privilege of living in neglect and dying neglected.

☙VIII☚

For the first few weeks after my arrival at the sanatorium, I was cared for by two attendants, one by day and one by night. I was still helpless, being unable to put my feet out of bed, much less upon the floor, and it was necessary that I be continually watched lest an impulse to walk should seize me. After a month or six weeks, however, I grew stronger, and from that time only one person was assigned to care for me. He was with me all day, and slept at night in the same room.

The earliest possible dismissal of one of my two attendants was expedient for the family purse; but such are the deficiencies in the prevailing treatment of the insane that relief in one direction often occasions evil in another. No sooner was the expense thus reduced than I was subjected to a detestable form of restraint which amounted to torture. To guard me at night while the remaining attendant slept, my hands were imprisoned in what is known as a "muff." A muff, innocent enough to the eyes of those who have never worn one, is in reality a relic of the Inquisition. It is an instrument of restraint which has been in use for centuries and even in many of our public and private institutions is still in use. The muff I wore was made of canvas, and differed in construction from a muff designed for the hands of fashion only in the inner partition, also of canvas, which separated my hands, but allowed them to overlap. At either

39

end was a strap which buckled tightly around the wrist and was locked.

The assistant physician, when he announced to me that I was to be subjected at night to this restraint, broke the news gently —so gently that I did not then know, nor did I guess for several months, why this thing was done to me. And thus it was that I drew deductions of my own which added not a little to my torture.

The gas jet in my room was situated at a distance, and stronger light was needed to find the keyholes and lock the muff when adjusted. Hence, an attendant was standing by with a lighted candle. Seating himself on the side of the bed, the physician said: "You won't try again to do what you did in New Haven, will you?" Now one may have done many things in a city where he has lived for a score of years, and it is not surprising that I failed to catch the meaning of the doctor's question. It was only after months of secret puzzling that I at last did discover his reference to my attempted suicide. But now the burning candle in the hands of the attendant, and a certain similarity between the doctor's name and the name of a man whose trial for arson I once attended out of idle curiosity, led me to imagine that in some way I had been connected with that crime. For some months I firmly believed I stood charged as an accomplice.

The putting on of the muff was the most humiliating incident of my life. The shaving of my legs and the wearing of the court-plaster brand of infamy had been humiliating, but those experiences had not overwhelmed my very heart as did this bitter ordeal. I resisted weakly, and, after the muff was adjusted and locked, for the first time since my mental collapse I wept. And I remember distinctly why I wept. The key that locked the muff unlocked in imagination the door of the home in New Haven which I believed I had disgraced—and seemed for a time to unlock my heart. Anguish beat my mind into a momentary sanity, and with a wholly sane emotion I keenly felt my imagined disgrace. My thoughts centred on my mother. Her (and other members of the family) I could plainly see at home in a state of dejection and despair over her imprisoned and heartless son. I wore the muff each night for several weeks, and for the first few nights the unhappy glimpse of a ruined home recurred and increased my sufferings.

It was not always as an instrument of restraint that the muff was employed. Frequently it was used as a means of discipline on account of supposed stubborn disobedience. Many times was I roughly overpowered by two attendants who locked my hands and coerced me to do whatever I had refused to do. My arms and hands were my only weapons of defence. My feet were still in plaster casts, and my back had been so severely injured as to necessitate my lying flat upon it most of the time. It was thus that these unequal fights were fought. And I had not even the satisfaction of tongue-lashing my oppressors, for I was practically speechless.

My attendants, like most others in such institutions, were incapable of understanding the operations of my mind, and what they could understand they would seldom tolerate. Yet they were not entirely to blame. They were simply carrying out to the letter orders received from the doctors.

To ask a patient in my condition to take a little medicated sugar seemed reasonable. But from my point of view my refusal was justifiable. That innocuous sugar disc to me seemed saturated with the blood of loved ones; and so much as to touch it was to shed their blood—perhaps on the very scaffold on which I was destined to die. For myself I cared little. I was anxious to die, and eagerly would I have taken the sugar disc had I had any reason to believe that it was deadly poison. The sooner I could die and be forgotten, the better for all with whom I had ever come in contact. To continue to live was simply to be the treacherous tool of unscrupulous detectives, eager to exterminate my innocent relatives and friends, if so their fame could be made secure in the annals of their craft.

But the thoughts associated with the taking of the medicine were seldom twice alike. If before taking it something happened to remind me of mother, father, some other relative, or a friend, I imagined that compliance would compromise, if not eventually destroy, that particular person. Who would not resist when meek acceptance would be a confession which would doom his own mother or father to prison, or ignominy, or death? It was for this that I was reviled, for this, subjected to cruel restraint.

They thought I was stubborn. In the strict sense of the word there is no such thing as a stubborn insane person. The truly stubborn men and women in the world are sane; and the fortunate prevalence of sanity may be approximately estimated by the preponderance of stubbornness in society at large. When one possessed of the power of recognizing his own errors continues to hold an unreasonable belief—that is stubbornness. But for a man bereft of reason to adhere to an idea which to him seems absolutely correct and true because he has been deprived of the means of detecting his error—that is not stubbornness. It is a symptom of his disease, and merits the indulgence of forbearance, if not genuine sympathy. Certainly the afflicted one deserves no punishment. As well punish with a blow the cheek that is disfigured by the mumps.

The attendant who was with me most of the time while I remained at the sanatorium was the kindly one already mentioned. Him I regarded, however, as a detective, or, rather, as two detectives, one of whom watched me by day, and the other —a perfect double—by night. He was an enemy, and his professed sympathy—which I now know was genuine—only made me hate him the more. As he was ignorant of the methods of treatment in vogue in hospitals for the insane, it was several weeks before he dared put in jeopardy his position by presuming to shield me against unwise orders of the doctors. But when at last he awoke to the situation, he repeatedly intervened in my behalf. More than once the doctor who was both owner and superintendent threatened to discharge him for alleged officiousness. But better judgment usually held the doctor's wrath in check, for he realized that not one attendant in a hundred was so competent.

Not only did the friendly attendant frequently exhibit more wisdom than the superintendent, but he also obeyed the dictates of a better conscience than that of his nominal superior, the assistant physician. On three occasions this man treated me with a signal lack of consideration, and in at least one instance he was vicious. When this latter incident occurred, I was both physically and mentally helpless. My feet were swollen and still in plaster bandages. I was all but mute, uttering only an occasional expletive when forced to perform acts against my will.

One morning Doctor No-name (he represents a type) entered my room.

"Good morning! How are you feeling?" he asked.

No answer.

"Aren't you feeling well?"

No answer.

"Why don't you talk?" he asked with irritation.

Still no answer, except perhaps a contemptuous look such as is so often the essence of eloquence. Suddenly, and without the slightest warning, as a petulant child locked in a room for disobedience might treat a pillow, he seized me by an arm and jerked me from the bed. It was fortunate that the bones of my ankles and feet, not yet thoroughly knitted, were not again injured. And this was the performance of the very man who had locked my hands in the muff, that I might not injure myself!

"Why don't you talk?" he again asked.

Though rather slow in replying, I will take pleasure in doing so by sending that doctor a copy of this book—my answer— if he will but send me his address.

It is not a pleasant duty to brand any physician for cruelty and incompetence, for the worst that ever lived has undoubtedly done many good deeds. But here is the type of man that has wrought havoc among the helpless insane. And the owner represented a type that has too long profited through the misfortunes of others. "Pay the price or put your relative in a public institution!" is the burden of his discordant song before commitment. "Pay or get out!" is his jarring refrain when satisfied that the family's resources are exhausted. I later learned that this grasping owner had bragged of making a profit of $98,000 in a single year. About twenty years later he left an estate of approximately $1,500,000. Some of the money, however, wrung from patients and their relatives in the past may yet benefit similar sufferers in the future, for, under the will of the owner, several hundred thousand dollars will eventually be available as an endowment for the institution.

ᴥIXᴥ

It was at the sanatorium that my ankles were finally restored to a semblance of their former utility. They were there subjected to a course of heroic treatment; but as today they permit me to walk, run, dance, and play tennis and golf, as do those who have never been crippled, my hours of torture endured under my first attempts to walk are almost pleasant to recall. About five months from the date of my injury I was allowed, or rather compelled, to place my feet on the floor and attempt to walk. My ankles were still swollen, absolutely without action, and acutely sensitive to the slightest pressure. From the time they were hurt until I again began to talk—two years later—I asked not one question as to the probability of my ever regaining the use of them. The fact was, I never expected to walk naturally again. The desire of the doctors to have me walk I believed to be inspired by the detectives, of whom, indeed, I supposed the doctor himself to be one. Had there been any confession to make, I am sure it would have been yielded under the stress of this ultimate torture. The million needle points which, just prior to my mental collapse, seemed to goad my brain, now centred their unwelcome attention on the soles of my feet. Had the floor been studded with minute stilettos my sufferings could hardly have been more intense. For several weeks assistance was necessary with each attempt to walk, and each attempt was an ordeal. Sweat stood in beads on either foot, wrung from my blood by agony. Believing that it would be only a question of time when I should be tried, condemned, and executed for some of my countless felonies, I thought that the attempt to prevent my continuing a cripple for the brief remainder of my days was prompted by anything but benevolence.

The superintendent would have proved himself more humane had he not peremptorily ordered my attendant to discontinue the use of a support which, until the plaster bandages were removed, had enabled me to keep my legs in a horizontal position when I sat up. His order was that I should put my legs down and keep them down, whether it hurt or not. The pain was of course intense when the blood again began to circulate freely through tissues long unused to its full pressure, and so evident was my distress that the attendant ignored the doctor's command and secretly favored me. He would remove the forbidden support for only a few minutes at a time, gradually lengthening the intervals until at last I was able to do without the support entirely. Before long and each day for several weeks I was forced at first to stagger and finally to walk across the room and back to the bed. The distance was increased as the pain diminished, until I was able to walk without more discomfort than a comparatively pleasant sensation of lameness. For at least two months after my feet first touched the floor I had to be carried up and downstairs, and for several months longer I went flat-footed.

Delusions of persecution—which include "delusions of self-reference"—though a source of annoyance while I was in an inactive state, annoyed and distressed me even more when I began to move about and was obliged to associate with other patients. To my mind, not only were the doctors and attendants detectives; each patient was a detective and the whole institution was a part of the Third Degree. Scarcely any remark was made in my presence that I could not twist into a cleverly veiled reference to myself. In each person I could see a resemblance to persons I had known, or to the principals or victims of the crimes with which I imagined myself charged. I refused to read; for to read veiled charges and fail to assert my innocence was to incriminate both myself and others. But I looked with longing glances upon all printed matter and, as my curiosity was continually piqued, this enforced abstinence grew to be well-nigh intolerable.

It became again necessary to the family purse that every possible saving be made. Accordingly, I was transferred from the main building, where I had a private room and a special attendant, to a ward where I was to mingle, under an aggregate sort of supervision, with fifteen or twenty other patients. Here I had no special attendant by day, though one slept in my room at night.

Of this ward I had heard alarming reports—and these from the lips of several attendants. I was, therefore, greatly disturbed at the proposed change. But, the transfer once accomplished, after a few days I really liked my new quarters better than the old. During the entire time I remained at the sanatorium I was more mentally alert than I gave evidence of being. But not until after my removal to this ward, where I was left alone for hours every day, did I dare to show my alertness. Here I even went so far on one occasion as to joke with the attendant in charge. He had been trying to persuade me to take a bath. I refused, mainly because I did not like the looks of the bath room, which, with its cement floor and central drain, resembled the room in which vehicles are washed in a modern stable. After all else had failed, the attendant tried the rôle of sympathizer.

"Now I know just how you feel," he said, "I can put myself in your place."

"Well, if you can, do it and take the bath yourself," was my retort.

The remark is brilliant by contrast with the dismal source from which it escaped. "Escaped" is the word; for the fear that

I should hasten my trial by exhibiting too great a gain in health, mental or physical, was already upon me; and it controlled much of my conduct during the succeeding months of depression.

Having now no special attendant, I spent many hours in my room, alone, but not absolutely alone, for somewhere the eye of a detective was evermore upon me. Comparative solitude, however, gave me courage; and soon I began to read, regardless of consequences. During the entire period of my depression, every publication seemed to have been written and printed for me, and me alone. Books, magazines, and newspapers seemed to be special editions. The fact that I well knew how inordinate would be the cost of such a procedure in no way shook my belief in it. Indeed, that I was costing my persecutors fabulous amounts of money was a source of secret satisfaction. My belief in special editions of newspapers was strengthened by items which seemed too trivial to warrant publication in any except editions issued for a special purpose. I recall a seemingly absurd advertisement, in which the phrase, "Green Bluefish," appeared. At the time I did not know that "green" was a term used to denote "fresh" or "unsalted."

During the earliest stages of my illness I had lost count of time, and the calendar did not right itself until the day when I largely regained my reason. Meanwhile, the date on each newspaper was, according to my reckoning, two weeks out of the way. This confirmed my belief in the special editions as a part of the Third Degree.

Most sane people think that no insane person can reason logically. But this is not so. Upon unreasonable premises I made most reasonable deductions, and that at the time when my mind was in its most disturbed condition. Had the newspapers which I read on the day which I supposed to be February 1st borne a January date, I might not then, for so long a time, have believed in special editions. Probably I should have inferred that the regular editions had been held back. But the newspapers I had were dated about two weeks *ahead*. Now if a sane person on February 1st receives a newspaper dated February 14th, he will be fully justified in thinking something wrong, either with the publication or with himself. But the shifted calendar which had planted itself in my mind meant as much to me as the true calendar does to any sane business man. During the seven hundred and ninety-eight days of depression I drew countless incorrect deductions. But, such as they were, they were deductions, and essentially the mental process was not other than that which takes places in a well-ordered mind.

My gradually increasing vitality, although it increased my fear of trial, impelled me to take new risks. I began to read not only newspapers, but also such books as were placed within my reach. Yet had they not been placed there, I should have gone without them, for I would never ask even for what I greatly desired and knew I could have for the asking.

Whatever love of literature I now have dates from this time, when I was a mental incompetent and confined in an institution. Lying on a shelf in my room was a book by George Eliot. For several days I cast longing glances at it and finally plucked up the courage to take nibbles now and then. These were so good that I grew bold and at last began openly to read the book. Its contents at the time made but little impression on my mind, but I enjoyed it. I read also some of Addison's essays; and had I been fortunate enough to have made myself familiar with these earlier in life, I might have been spared the delusion that I could detect, in many passages, the altering hand of my persecutors.

The friendly attendant, from whom I was now separated, tried to send his favors after me into my new quarters. At first he came in person to see me, but the superintendent soon forbade that, and also ordered him not to communicate with me in any way. It was this disagreement, and others naturally arising between such a doctor and such an attendant, that soon brought about the discharge of the latter. But "discharge" is hardly the word, for he had become disgusted with the institution, and had remained so long only because of his interest in me. Upon leaving, he informed the owner that he would soon cause my removal from the institution. This he did. I left the sanatorium in March, 1901, and remained for three months in the home of this kindly fellow, who lived with a grandmother and an aunt in Wallingford, a town not far from New Haven.

It is not to be inferred that I entertained any affection for my friendly keeper. I continued to regard him as an enemy; and my life at his home became a monotonous round of displeasure. I took my three meals a day. I would sit listlessly for hours at a time in the house. Daily I went out—accompanied, of course —for short walks about the town. These were not enjoyable. I believed everybody was familiar with my black record and expected me to be put to death. Indeed, I wondered why passers-by did not revile or even stone me. Once I was sure I heard a little girl call me "Traitor!" That, I believe, was my last "false voice," but it made such an impression that I can even now recall vividly the appearance of that dreadful child. It was not surprising that a piece of rope, old and frayed, which someone had carelessly thrown on a hedge by a cemetery that I sometimes passed, had for me great significance.

During these three months I again refused to read books, though within my reach, but I sometimes read newspapers. Still I would not speak, except under some unusual stress of emotion. The only time I took the initiative in this regard while living in the home of my attendant was on a bitterly cold and snowy day when I had the temerity to tell him that the wind had blown the blanket from a horse that had been standing for a long time in front of the house. The owner had come inside to transact some business with my attendant's relatives. In appearance he reminded me of the uncle to whom this book is dedicated. I imagined the mysterious caller was impersonating him and, by one of my curious mental processes, I deduced that it was incumbent on me to do for the dumb beast outside what I knew my uncle would have done had he been aware of its plight. My reputation for decency of feeling I believed to be gone forever; but I could not bear, in this situation, to be unworthy of my uncle, who, among those who knew him, was famous for his kindliness and humanity.

My attendant and his relatives were very kind and very patient, for I was still intractable. But their efforts to make me comfortable, so far as they had any effect, made keener my desire to kill myself. I shrank from death; but I preferred to die by my own hand and take the blame for it, rather than to be executed and bring lasting disgrace on my family, friends, and, I may add with truth, on Yale. For I reasoned that parents throughout the country would withhold their sons from a university which numbered among its graduates such a despicable being. But from any tragic act I was providentially restrained by the very delusion which gave birth to the desire—in a way which signally appeared on a later and, to me, a memorable day.

X

I am in a position not unlike that of a man whose obituary notice has appeared prematurely. Few have ever had a better opportunity than I to test the affection of their relatives and friends. That mine did their duty and did it willingly is naturally a constant source of satisfaction to me. Indeed, I believe that this unbroken record of devotion is one of the factors which eventually made it possible for me to take up again my duties in the social and business world, with a comfortable feeling of continuity. I can, indeed, now view my past in as matter-of-fact a way as do those whose lives have been uniformly uneventful.

As I have seen scores of patients neglected by their relatives —a neglect which they resent and often brood upon—my sense of gratitude is the livelier, and especially so because of the difficulty with which friendly intercourse with me was maintained during two of the three years I was ill. Relatives and friends frequently called to see me. True, these calls were trying for all concerned. I spoke to none, not even to my mother and father. For, though they all appeared about as they used to, I was able to detect some slight difference in look or gesture or intonation of voice, and this was enough to confirm my belief that they were impersonators, engaged in a conspiracy, not merely to entrap me, but to incriminate those whom they impersonated. It is not strange, then, that I refused to say anything to them, or to permit them to come near me. To have kissed the woman who was my mother, but whom I believed to be a federal conspirator, would have been an act of betrayal. These interviews were much harder for my relatives and friends than for me. But even for me they were ordeals; and though I suffered less at these moments than my callers, my sum of suffering was greater, for I was constantly anticipating these unwelcome, but eventually beneficial, visitations.

Suppose my relatives and friends had held aloof during this apparently hopeless period, what to-day would be my feelings toward them? Let others answer. For over two years I considered all letters forgeries. Yet the day came when I convinced myself of their genuineness and the genuineness of the love of those who sent them. Perhaps persons who have relatives among the more than a quarter of a million patients in institutions in this country today will find some comfort in this fact. To be on the safe and humane side, let every relative and friend of persons so afflicted remember the Golden Rule, which has never been suspended with respect to the insane. Go to see them, treat them sanely, write to them, keep them informed about the home circle; let not your devotion flag, nor accept any repulse.

The consensus now was that my condition was unlikely ever to improve, and the question of my commitment to some institution where incurable cases could be cared for came up for decision. While it was being considered, my attendant kept assuring me that it would be unnecessary to commit me to an institution if I would but show some improvement. So he repeatedly suggested that I go to New Haven and spend a day at home. At this time, it will be recalled, I was all but mute, so, being unable to beguile me into speech, the attendant one morning laid out for my use a more fashionable shirt than I usually wore, telling me to put it on if I wished to make the visit. That day it took me an unusually long time to dress, but in the end I put on the designated garment. Thus did one part of my brain outwit another.

I simply chose the less of two evils. The greater was to find myself again committed to an institution. Nothing else would have induced me to go to New Haven. I did not wish to go. To my best knowledge and belief, I had no home there, nor did I have any relatives or friends who would greet me upon my return. How could they, if still free, even approach me while I was surrounded by detectives? Then, too, I had a lurking suspicion that my attendant's offer was made in the belief that I would not dare accept it. By taking him at his word, I knew that I should at least have an opportunity to test the truth of many of his statements regarding my old home. Life had become insupportable; and back of my consent to make this experimental visit was a willingness to beard the detectives in their own den, regardless of consequences. With these and many other reflections I started for the train. The events of the journey which followed are of no moment. We soon reached the New Haven station; and, as I had expected, no relative or friend was there to greet us. This apparent indifference seemed to support my suspicion that my attendant had not told me the truth; but I found little satisfaction in uncovering his deceit, for the more of a liar I proved him to be, the worse would be my plight. We walked to the front of the station and stood there for almost half an hour. The unfortunate, but perfectly natural, wording of a question caused the delay.

"Well, shall we go home?" my attendant said.

How could I say, "Yes"? I had no home. I feel sure I should finally have said, "No," had he continued to put the question in that form. Consciously or unconsciously, however, he altered it. "Shall we go to 30 Trumbull Street?" That was what I had been waiting for. Certainly I would go to the house designated by that number. I had come to New Haven to see that house;

and I had just a faint hope that its appearance and the appearance of its occupants might prove convincing.

At home my visit came as a complete surprise. I could not believe that my relatives—if they were relatives—had not been informed of my presence in the city, and their words and actions upon my arrival confirmed my suspicion and extinguished the faint hope I had briefly cherished. My hosts were simply the same old persecutors with whom I had already had too much to do. Soon after my arrival, dinner was served. I sat at my old place at the table, and secretly admired the skill with which he who asked the blessing imitated the language and the well-remembered intonation of my father's voice. But alas for the family!—I imagined my relatives banished and languishing in prison, and the old home confiscated by the government!

❧XI❧

Though my few hours at home failed to prove that I did not belong in an institution, it served one good purpose. Certain relatives who had objected to my commitment now agreed that there was no alternative, and, accordingly, my eldest brother caused himself to be appointed my conservator. He had long favored taking such action, but other relatives had counseled delay. They had been deterred by that inbred dread of seeing a member of the family branded by law as a mental incompetent, and, to a degree, stigmatized by the prevailing unwarranted attitude of the public toward mental illness and the institutions in which mental cases are treated. The very thought was repellent; and a mistaken sense of duty—and perhaps a suggestion of pride—led them to wish me out of such an institution as long as possible.

Though at the time I dreaded commitment, it was the best possible thing that could befall me. To be, as I was, in the world but not of it, was exasperating. The constant friction that is inevitable under such conditions—conditions such as existed for me in the home of my attendant—can only aggravate the mental disturbance. Especially is this true of those laboring under delusions of persecution. Such delusions multiply with the complexity of the life led. It is the even-going routine of institutional life which affords the indispensable quieting effect—provided that routine is well ordered, and not defeated by annoyances imposed by ignorant or indifferent doctors and attendants.

My commitment occurred on June 11th, 1901. The institution to which I was committed was a chartered, private institution, but not run for personal profit. It was considered one of the best of its kind in the country and was pleasantly situated. Though the view was a restricted one, a vast expanse of lawn, surrounded by groups of trees, like patches of primeval forest, gave the place an atmosphere which was not without its remedial effect. My quarters were comfortable, and after a little time I adjusted myself to my new environment.

Breakfast was served about half-past seven, though the hour varied somewhat according to the season—earlier in summer and later in winter. In the spring, summer, and autumn, when the weather was favorable, those able to go out of doors were taken after breakfast for walks within the grounds, or were allowed to roam about the lawn and sit under the trees, where they remained for an hour or two at a time. Dinner was usually served shortly after noon, and then the active patients were again taken out of doors, where they remained an hour or two doing much as they pleased, but under watchful eyes. About half-past three they returned to their respective wards, there to remain until the next day—except those who cared to attend the religious service which was held almost every afternoon in an endowed chapel.

In all institutions those confined in different kinds of wards go to bed at different hours. The patients in the best wards retire at nine or ten o'clock. Those in the wards where more troublesome cases are treated go to bed usually at seven or eight o'clock. I, while undergoing treatment, have retired at all hours, so that I am in the better position to describe the mysteries of what is, in a way, one of the greatest secret societies in the world. I soon became accustomed to the rather agreeable routine, and had I not been burdened with the delusions which held me a prisoner of the police, and kept me a stranger to my old world, I should have been able to enjoy a comparatively happy existence in spite of it all.

This new feeling of comparative contentment had not been brought about by any marked improvement in health. It was due directly and entirely to an environment more nearly in tune with my ill-tuned mind. While surrounded by sane people my mental inferiority had been painfully apparent to me, as well as to others. Here a feeling of superiority easily asserted itself, for many of my associates were, to my mind, vastly inferior to myself. But this stimulus did not affect me at once. For several weeks I believed the institution to be peopled by detectives, feigning insanity. The government was still operating the Third Degree, only on a grander scale. Nevertheless, I did soon come to the conclusion that the institution was what it purported to be —still cherishing the idea, however, that certain patients and attachés were detectives.

For a while after my arrival I again abandoned my new-found reading habit. But as I became accustomed to my surroundings I grew bolder and resumed the reading of newspapers and such books as were at hand. There was a bookcase in the ward, filled with old numbers of standard English periodicals; among them: *Westminster Review, Edinburgh Review, London Quarterly,* and *Blackwood's.* There were also copies of *Harper's* and *The Atlantic Monthly,* dated a generation or more before my first reading days. Indeed, some of the reviews were over fifty years old. But I had to read their heavy contents or go without reading, for I would not yet ask even for a thing I ardently desired. In the room of one of the patients were thirty or forty books belonging to him. Time and again I walked by his door and cast longing glances at those books, which at first I had not the courage to ask for or to take. But during the summer, about the time I was getting desperate, I finally managed to summon enough courage to take them surreptitiously. It was usually while the owner of these books was attending the daily service in the chapel that his library became a circulating one.

The contents of the books I read made perhaps a deeper impression on my memory than most books make on the minds of normal readers. To assure myself of the fact, I have since reread "The Scarlet Letter," and I recognize it as an old friend. The first part of the story, however, wherein Hawthorne describes his work as a Custom House official and portrays his literary personality, seems to have made scarcely any impression. This I attribute to my utter lack of interest at that time in writers and their methods. I then had no desire to write a book, nor any thought of ever doing so.

Letters I looked upon with suspicion. I never read them at the time they were received. I would not even open them; but generally, after a week or sometimes a month, I would secretly open and read them—forgeries of the detectives.

I still refused to speak, and exhibited physical activity only when the patients were taken out of doors. For hours I would sit reading books or newspapers, or apparently doing nothing. But my mind was in an active state and very sensitive. As the event proved, almost everything done or said within the range of my senses was making indelible impressions, though these at the time were frequently of such a character that I experienced great difficulty in trying to recall incidents which I thought I might find useful at the time of my appearance in court.

My ankles had not regained anything like their former strength. It hurt to walk. For months I continued to go flat-footed. I could not sustain my weight with heels lifted from the floor. In going downstairs I had to place my insteps on the edge of each step, or go one step at a time, like a child. Believing that the detectives were pampering me into prime condition, as a butcher fattens a beast for slaughter, I deliberately made myself out much weaker than I really was; and not a little of my inactivity was due to a desire to prolong my fairly comfortable existence, by deferring as long as possible the day of trial and conspicuous disgrace.

But each day still had its distressing incidents. Whenever the attendants were wanted at the office, an electric bell was rung. During the fourteen months that I remained in this hospital in a depressed condition, the bell in my ward rang several hundred times. Never did it fail to send through me a mild shock of terror, for I imagined that at last the hour had struck for my transportation to the scene of trial. Relatives and friends would be brought to the ward—heralded, of course, by a warning bell —and short interviews would be held in my room, during which the visitors had to do all the talking. My eldest brother, whom I shall refer to hereafter as my conservator, called often. He seldom failed to use one phrase which worried me.

"You are looking better and getting stronger," he would say. "We shall straighten you out yet."

To be "straightened out" was an ambiguous phrase which might refer to the end of the hangman's rope or to a fatal electric shock.

I preferred to be let alone, and the assistant physician in charge of my case, after several ineffectual attempts to engage me in conversation, humored my persistent taciturnity. For more than a year his only remarks to me were occasional conventional salutations. Subsequent events have led me to doubt the wisdom of his policy.

For one year no further attention was paid to me than to see that I had three meals a day, the requisite number of baths, and a sufficient amount of exercise. I was, however, occasionally urged by an attendant to write a letter to some relative, but that, of course, I refused to do. As I shall have many hard things to say about attendants in general, I take pleasure in testifying that, so long as I remained in a passive condition, those at this institution were kind, and at times even thoughtful. But there came a time when diplomatic relations with doctors and attendants became so strained that war promptly ensued.

It was no doubt upon the gradual, but sure improvement in my physical condition that the doctors were relying for my eventual return to normality. They were not without some warrant for this. In a way I had become less suspicious, but my increased confidence was due as much to an increasing indifference to my fate as to an improvement in health. And there were other signs of improved mental vigor. I was still watchful, however, for a chance to end my life, and, but for a series of fortunate circumstances, I do not doubt that my choice of evils would have found tragic expression in an overt act.

Having convinced myself that most of my associates were really insane, and therefore (as I believed) disqualified as competent witnesses in a court of law, I would occasionally engage in conversation with a few whose evident incompetency seemed to make them safe confidants. One, a man who during his life had more than once been committed to an institution, took a very evident interest in me and persisted in talking to me, often much against my will. His persistent inquisitiveness seemed to support his own statement that he had formerly been a successful life-insurance agent. He finally gained my confidence to such a degree that months before I finally began to talk to others I permitted myself to converse frequently with him—but only when we were so situated as to escape observation. I would talk to him on almost any subject, but would not speak about myself. At length, however, his admirable persistence overcame my reticence. During a conversation held in June, 1902, he abruptly said, "Why you are kept here I cannot understand. Apparently you are as sane as anyone. You have never made any but sensible remarks to me." Now for weeks I had been waiting for a chance to tell this man my very thoughts. I had come to believe him a true friend who would not betray me.

"If I should tell you some things which you apparently don't know, you would understand why I am held here," I said.

"Well, tell me," he urged.

"Will you promise not to repeat my statements to any one else?"

"I promise not to say a word."

"Well," I remarked, "you have seen certain persons who have come here, professing to be relatives of mine."

"Yes, and they are your relatives, aren't they?"

"They look like my relatives, but they're not," was my reply.

My inquisitive friend burst into laughter and said, "Well, if you mean *that,* I shall have to take back what I just said. You are really the craziest person I have ever met, and I have met several."

"You will think differently some day," I replied; for I believed that when my trial should occur, he would appreciate the significance of my remark. I did not tell him that I believed these callers to be detectives; nor did I hint that I thought myself in the hands of the police.

Meanwhile, during July and August, 1902, I redoubled my activity in devising suicidal schemes; for I now thought my physical condition satisfactory to my enemies, and was sure that my trial could not be postponed beyond the next opening of the courts in September. I even went so far as to talk to one of the attendants, a medical student, who during the summer worked as an attendant at the hospital. I approached him artfully. First I asked him to procure from the library for me "The Scarlet Letter," "The House of Seven Gables," and other books; then I talked medicine and finally asked him to lend me a textbook on anatomy which I knew he had in his possession. This he did, cautioning me not to let anyone know that he had done so. The book once secured, I lost no time in examining that part which described the heart, its functions, and especially its exact position in the body. I had scarcely begun to read when the young man returned and took the book from me, giving as his reason that an attendant had no right to let a patient read a medical work. Maybe his change of heart was providential.

As is usual in these institutions, all knives, forks, and other articles that might be used by a patient for a dangerous purpose were counted by the attendants after each meal. This I knew, and the knowledge had a deterrent effect. I dared not take one. Though I might at any time during the night have hanged myself, that method did not appeal to me, and I kept it in mind only as a last resort. To get possession of some sharp dagger-like instrument which I could plunge into my heart at a moment's notice—this was my consuming desire. With such a weapon I felt that I could, when the crisis came, rob the detectives of their victory. During the summer months an employé spent his entire time mowing the lawn with a large horse-drawn machine. This, when not in use, was often left outdoors. Upon it was a square wooden box, containing certain necessary tools, among them a sharp spike-like instrument, used to clean the oil-holes when they became clogged. This bit of steel was five or six inches long, and was shaped like a pencil. For at least three months, I seldom went out of doors that I did not go with the intention of purloining that steel spike. I intended then to keep it in my room against the day of my anticipated transfer to jail.

It was now that my delusions protected me from the very fate they had induced me to court. For had I not believed that the eye of a detective was on me every moment, I could have taken that spike a score of times. Often, when it was not in use, I walked to the lawnmower and even laid my hand upon the tool-box. But I dared not open it. My feelings were much like those of Pandora about a certain other box. In my case, however, the box upon which I looked with longing had Hope without, and not within. Instinctively, perhaps, I realized this, for I did not lift the lid.

One day, as the patients were returning to their wards, I saw, lying directly in my path (I could even now point out the spot), the coveted weapon. Never have I seen anything that I wanted more. To have stooped and picked it up without detection would have been easy; and had I known, as I know now, that it had been carelessly dropped there, nothing could have prevented me from doing so and perhaps using it with fatal effect. But I believed it had been placed there deliberately and as a test, by those who had divined my suicidal purpose. The eye of the imagined detective, which, I am inclined to believe, and like to believe, was the eye of the real God, was upon me; and though I stepped directly over it, I did not pick up that thing of death.

☙ XII ❧

When I had decided that my chance for securing the little stiletto spike was very uncertain, I at once busied myself with plans which were designed to bring about my death by drowning. There was in the ward a large bath tub. Access to it could be had at any time, except from the hour of nine (when the patients were locked in their rooms for the night) until the following morning. How to reach it during the night was the problem which confronted me. The attendant in charge was supposed to see that each patient was in his room before his door was locked. As it rarely happened that the patients were not in their rooms at the appointed time, the attendants naturally grew careless, and often locked a door without looking in. "Good night"—a salutation usually devoid of sentiment—might, or might not, elicit a response, and the absence of a response would not tend to arouse suspicion—especially in a case like mine, for I would sometimes say "good night," but more often not.

My simple and easy plan was to hide behind a piece of furniture in the corridor and there remain until the attendant had locked the doors of the rooms and gone to bed. I had even advanced so far in my plan as to select a convenient nook within twenty feet of my own room. Should the attendant, when about to lock the door, discover my absence, I should, of course, immediately reveal my hiding-place by leaving it; and it would have been an easy matter to convince him that I had done the thing as a test of his own vigilance. On the other hand, if I escaped discovery, I should then have nine hours at my disposal with little fear of interruption. True, the night watch passed through the ward once every hour. But death by drowning requires a time no longer than that necessary to boil an egg. I had even calculated how long it would take to fill the tub with water. To make sure of a fatal result, I had secreted a piece of wire which I intended so to use that my head, once under water, could by no possibility be raised above the surface in the inevitable death struggle.

I have said that I did not desire death; nor did I. Had the supposed detectives been able to convince me that they would keep their word, I would willingly have signed an agreement stipulating on my side that I must live the rest of my life in confinement, and on theirs that I should never undergo a trial for crime.

Fortunately, during these dismal preparations, I had not lost interest in other schemes which probably saved my life. In these the fellow-patient who had won my confidence played the rôle of my own private detective. That he and I could defeat the combined forces arrayed against me hardly seemed probable, but the seeming impossibility of so doing only lent zest to the undertaking. My friend, who, of course, did not realize that he was engaged in combat with the Secret Service, was allowed to go where he pleased within the limits of the city where the hospital was situated. Accordingly I determined to enlist his services. It was during July that, at my suggestion, he tried to procure copies of certain New Haven newspapers, of the date of my attempted suicide and the several dates immediately following. My purpose was to learn what motive had been ascribed to my suicidal act. I felt sure that the papers would contain at least hints as to the nature of the criminal charges against me. But my purpose I did not disclose to my friend. In due time he reported that no copies for the given dates were to be had. So *that* quest proved fruitless, and I attributed the failure to the superior strategy of the enemy.

Meanwhile, my friend had not stopped trying to convince me that my apparent relatives were not spurious; so one day I said to him: "If my relatives still live in New Haven, their addresses must be in the latest New Haven Directory. Here is a list containing the names and former addresses of my father, brother and uncle. These were their addresses in 1900. To-morrow, when you go out, please see whether they appear in the New Haven Directory for 1902. These persons who present themselves to me as relatives pretend to live at these addresses. If they speak the truth, the 1902 Directory will corroborate them. I shall then have hope that a letter sent to any one of these addresses will reach relatives—and surely some attention will be paid to it."

The next day, my own good detective went to a local publishing house where directories of important cities throughout the country could be consulted. Shortly after he went upon this errand, my conservator appeared. He found me walking about the lawn. At his suggestion we sat down. Bold in the assurance that I could kill myself before the crisis came, I talked with him freely, replying to many of his questions and asking several. My conservator, who did not know that I doubted his identity, commented with manifest pleasure on my new-found readiness to talk. He would have been less pleased, however, had he been able to read my mind.

Shortly after my conservator's departure, my fellow-patient returned and informed me that the latest New Haven Directory contained the names and addresses I had given him. This information, though it did not prove that my morning caller was no detective, did not convince me that my real brother still lived where he did when I left New Haven, two years earlier. Now that my delusions were growing weaker, my returning reason enabled me to construct the ingenious scheme which, I believe, saved my life; for, had I not largely regained my reason *when I did,* I am inclined to believe that my distraught mind would have destroyed itself and me, before it could have been restored by the slow process of returning health.

A few hours after my own private detective had given me the information I so much desired, I wrote the first letter I had written in twenty-six months. As letters go, it is in a class by itself. I dared not ask for ink, so I wrote with a lead pencil. Another fellow-patient in whom I had confidence, at my request, addressed the envelope; but he was not in the secret of its contents. This was an added precaution, for I thought the Secret Service men might have found out that I had a detective of my own and would confiscate any letters addressed by him or me. The next morning, *my* "detective" mailed the letter. That letter I still have, and I treasure it as any innocent man condemned to death would treasure a pardon. It should convince the reader that sometimes a mentally disordered person, even one suffering from many delusions, can think and write clearly. An exact copy of this—the most important letter I ever expect to be called upon to write—is here presented:

AUGUST 29, 1902.

DEAR GEORGE:

On last Wednesday morning a person who claimed to be George M. Beers of New Haven, Ct., clerk in the Director's Office of the Sheffield Scientific School and a brother of mine, called to see me.

Perhaps what he said was true, but after the events of the last two years I find myself inclined to doubt the truth of everything that is told me. He said that he would come and see me again sometime next week, and I am sending you this letter in order that you may bring it with you as a passport, provided you *are* the one who was here on Wednesday.

If you did not call as stated please say nothing about this letter to anyone, and when your double arrives, I'll tell him what I think of him. Would send other messages, but while things seems as they do at present it is impossible. Have had someone else address envelope for fear letter might be held up on the way.

Yours,
CLIFFORD W. B.

Though I felt reasonably confident that this message would reach my brother, I was by no means certain. I was sure, however, that, should he receive it, under no circumstances would he turn it over to anyone hostile to myself. When I wrote the words: "Dear George," my feeling was much like that of a child who sends a letter to Santa Claus after his childish faith has been shaken. Like the skeptical child, I felt there was nothing to lose, but everything to gain. "Yours" fully expressed such affection for relatives as I was then capable of—for the belief that I had disgraced, perhaps destroyed, my family prompted me to forbear to use the family name in the signature.

The thought that I might soon get in touch with my old world did not excite me. I had not much faith anyway that I was to re-establish former relations with it, and what little faith I had was all but destroyed on the morning of August 30th, 1902, when a short message, written on a slip of paper, reached me by the hand of an attendant. It informed me that my conservator would call that afternoon. I thought it a lie. I felt that any brother of mine would have taken the pains to send a letter in reply to the first I had written him in over two years. The thought that there had not been time for him to do so and that this message must have arrived by telephone did not then occur to me. What I believed was that my own letter had been confiscated. I asked one of the doctors to swear on his honor that it really was my own brother who was coming to see me. This he did. But abnormal suspicion robbed all men in my sight of whatever honor they may have had, and I was not fully re-assured.

In the afternoon, as usual, the patients were taken out of doors, I among them. I wandered about the lawn and cast fre-quent and expectant glances toward the gate, through which I believed my anticipated visitor would soon pass. In less than an hour he appeared. I first caught sight of him about three hundred feet away, and, impelled more by curiosity than hope, I advanced to meet him. "I wonder what the lie will be this time," was the gist of my thoughts.

The person approaching me was indeed the counterpart of my brother as I remembered him. Yet he was no more my brother than he had been at any time during the preceding two years. He was still a detective. Such he was when I shook his hand. As soon as that ceremony was over, he drew forth a leather pocketbook. I instantly recognized it as one I myself had carried for several years prior to the time I was taken ill in 1900. It was from this that he took my recent letter.

"Here's my passport," he said.

"It's a good thing you brought it," I replied, as I glanced at it and again shook his hand—this time the hand of my own brother.

"Don't you want to read it?" he asked.

"There is no need of that. I am convinced."

After my long journey of exploration in the jungle of a tangled imagination, a journey which finally ended in my find-ing the person for whom I had long searched, my behavior differed very little from that of a great explorer who, full of doubt after a long and perilous trip through real jungles, found the man he sought and, grasping his hand, greeted him with the simple and historic words, "Dr. Livingstone, I presume?"

The very instant I caught sight of my letter in the hands of my brother, all was changed. The thousands of false impressions recorded during the seven hundred and ninety-eight days of my depression seemed at once to correct themselves. Untruth became Truth. A large part of what was once my old world was again mine. To me, at least, my mind seemed to have found itself, for the gigantic web of false beliefs in which it had been all but hopelessly enmeshed I now immediately recognized as a snare of delusions. That the Gordian knot of mental torture should be cut and swept away by the mere glance of a willing eye is like a miracle. Not a few patients, however, suffering from certain forms of mental disorder, regain a high degree of insight into their mental condition in what might be termed a flash of divine enlightenment. Though insight regained seemingly in an instant is a most encouraging symptom, power to reason normally on all subjects cannot, of course, be so promptly recovered. My new power to reason correctly on some subjects simply marked the transition from depression, one phase of my disorder, to elation, another phase of it. Medically speaking, I was as mentally disordered as before—yet I was happy!

My memory during depression may be likened to a photographic film, seven hundred and ninety-eight days long. Each impression seems to have been made in a negative way and then, in a fraction of a second, miraculously developed and made positive. Of hundreds of impressions made during that depressed period I had not before been conscious, but from the moment my mind, if not my full reason, found itself, they stood out vividly. Not only so, but other impressions registered during earlier years became clearer. Since that August 30th, which I regard as my second birthday (my first was on the 30th of another month), my mind has exhibited qualities which, prior to that time, were so latent as to be scarcely distinguishable. As a result, I find myself able to do desirable things I never before dreamed of doing—the writing of this book is one of them.

Yet had I failed to convince myself on August 30th, when

my brother came to see me, that he was no spy, I am almost sure that I should have compassed my own destruction within the following ten days, for the next month, I believed, was the fatal one of opening courts. You will recall that it was death by drowning that impended. I liken my salvation itself to a prolonged process of drowning. Thousands of minutes of the seven hundred and ninety-eight days—and there were over one million of them, during which I had been borne down by intolerably burdensome delusions—were, I imagine, much like the last minutes of consciousness experienced by persons who drown. Many who have narrowly escaped that fate can testify to the vividness with which good and bad impressions of their entire life rush through their confused minds, and hold them in a grip of terror until a kind unconsciousness envelops them. Such had been many of my moments. But the only unconsciousness which had deadened my sensibilities during these two despondent years was that of sleep itself. Though I slept fairly well most of the time, mine was seldom a dreamless sleep. Many of my dreams were, if anything, harder to bear than my delusions of the day, for what little reason I had was absolutely suspended in sleep. Almost every night my brain was at battledore and shuttlecock with weird thoughts. And if not all my dreams were terrifying, this fact seemed to be only because a perverted and perverse Reason, in order that its possessor might not lose the capacity for suffering, knew how to keep Hope alive with visions which supplied the contrast necessary for keen appreciation.

No man can be born again, but I believe I came as near it as ever a man did. To leave behind what was in reality a hell, and immediately have this good green earth revealed in more glory than most men ever see it, was one of the compensating privileges which make me feel that my suffering was worth while.

I have already described the peculiar sensation which assailed me when, in June, 1900, I lost my reason. At that time my brain felt as though pricked by a million needles at white heat. On this August 30th, 1902, shortly after largely regaining my reason, I had another most distinct sensation in the brain. It started under my brow and gradually spread until the entire surface was affected. The throes of a dying Reason had been torture. The sensations felt as my dead Reason was reborn were delightful. It seemed as though the refreshing breath of some kind Goddess of Wisdom were being blown gently against the surface of my brain. It was a sensation not unlike that produced by a menthol pencil rubbed ever so gently over a fevered brow. So delicate, so crisp and exhilarating was it that words fail me in my attempt to describe it. Few, if any, experiences can be more delightful. If the exaltation produced by some drugs is anything like it, I can easily understand how and why certain pernicious habits enslave those who contract them. For me, however, this experience was liberation, not enslavement.

৵XIIIঌ

After two years of silence I found it no easy matter to carry on with my brother a sustained conversation. So weak were my vocal cords from lack of use that every few minutes I must either rest or whisper. And upon pursing my lips I found myself unable to whistle, notwithstanding the popular belief, drawn from vague memories of small-boyhood, that this art is instinctive. Those who all their lives have talked at will cannot possibly appreciate the enjoyment I found in using my regained power of speech. Reluctantly I returned to the ward; but not until my brother had left for home, laden with so much of my conversation that it took most of his leisure for the next two days to tell the family what I had said in two hours.

During the first few hours I seemed virtually normal. I had none of the delusions which had previously oppressed me; nor had I yet developed any of the expansive ideas, or delusions of grandeur, which soon began to crowd in upon me. So normal did I appear while talking to my brother that he thought I should be able to return home in a few weeks; and, needless to say, I agreed with him. But the pendulum, as it were, had swung too far. The human brain is too complex a mechanism to admit of any such complete readjustment in an instant. It is said to be composed of several million cells; and, that fact granted, it seems safe to say that every day, perhaps every hour,

74

hundreds of thousands of the cells of my brain were now being brought into a state of renewed activity. Comparatively sane and able to recognize the important truths of life, I was yet insane as to many of its practical details. Judgment being King of the Realm of Thought, it was not surprising that my judgment failed often to decide correctly the many questions presented to it by its abnormally communicative subjects. At first I seemed to live in a second childhood. I did with delight many things which I had first learned to do as a child—the more so as it had been necessary for me to learn again to eat and walk, and now to talk. I had much lost time to make up; and for a while my sole ambition seemed to be to utter as many thousand words a day as possible. My fellow-patients who for fourteen months had seen me walk about in silence—a silence so profound and inexorable that I would seldom heed their friendly salutations—were naturally surprised to see me in my new mood of unrestrained loquacity and irrepressible good humor. In short, I had come into that abnormal condition which is known to psychiatrists as elation.

For several weeks I believe I did not sleep more than two or three hours a night. Such was my state of elation, however, that all signs of fatigue were entirely absent; and the sustained and abnormal mental and physical activity in which I then indulged has left on my memory no other than a series of very pleasant impressions. Though based on fancy, the delights of some forms of mental disorder are real. Few, if any, sane persons would care to test the matter at so great a price; but those familiar with the "Letters of Charles Lamb" must know that Lamb, himself, underwent treatment for mental disease. In a letter to Coleridge, dated June 10th, 1796, he says: "At some future time I will amuse you with an account, as full as my memory will permit, of the strange turns my frenzy took. I look back upon it at times with a gloomy kind of envy; for, while it lasted, I had many, many hours of pure happiness. Dream not, Coleridge, of having tasted all the grandeur of wildness of Fancy till you have gone mad! All now seems to me vapid, comparatively so!"

As for me, the very first night vast but vague humanitarian projects began joyously to shape themselves in my mind. My garden of thoughts seemed filled with flowers which might properly be likened to the quick-blowing night-blooming cereus —that Delusion of Grandeur of all flowering plants that thinks itself prodigal enough if it but unmask its beauty to the moon! Few of my bold fancies, however, were of so fugitive and chaste a splendor.

The religious instinct is found in primitive man. It is not strange, therefore, that at this time the religious side of my nature was the first to display compelling activity. Whether or not this was due to my rescue from a living death, and my immediate appreciation of God's goodness, both to me and to those faithful relatives who had done all the praying during the preceding two years—this I cannot say. But the fact stands out, that, whereas I had, while depressed, attached a sinister signifi- cance to everything done or said in my presence, I now inter- preted the most trifling incidents as messages from God. The day after this transition I attended church. It was the first service in over two years which I had not attended against my will. The reading of a psalm—the 45th—made a lasting impression upon me, and the interpretation which I placed upon it fur- nishes the key to my attitude during the first weeks of elation. It seemed to me a direct message from Heaven.

The minister began: "My heart is inditing a good matter: I speak of the things which I have made touching the king: my tongue is the pen of a ready writer."—Whose heart but mine? And the things indited—what were they but the humanitarian projects which had blossomed in my garden of thoughts over night? When, a few days later, I found myself writing very long letters with unwonted facility, I became convinced that my tongue was to prove itself "the pen of a ready writer." Indeed, to these prophetic words I trace the inception of an irresistible desire, of which this book is the first fruit.

"Thou art fairer than the children of men; grace is poured into thy lips:" was the verse next read (by myself and the congregation), to which the minister responded, "Therefore God hath blessed thee for ever."—"Surely, I have been selected as the instrument wherewith great reforms shall be effected." was my thought. (All is grist that comes to the mill of a mind in elation—then even divine encomiums seem not undeserved.)

"Gird thy sword upon thy thigh, O most mighty, with thy glory and thy majesty"—a command to fight. "And in thy majesty ride prosperously because of truth and meekness and righteousness;" replied the minister. "And thy right hand shall teach thee terrible things,"—was another response. That I could speak the truth, I knew. "Meekness" I could not associate with myself, except that during the preceding two years I had suffered many indignities without open resentment. That my right hand with a pen should teach me terrible things—how to fight for reform—I firmly believed.

"Thine arrows are sharp in the heart of the King's enemies, whereby the people fall under thee," quoth the minister. Yes, my tongue could be as sharp as an arrow, and I should be able to stand up against those who should stand in the way of reform. Again: "Thou lovest righteousness and hatest wickedness. Therefore God, thy God, hath anointed thee with the oil of gladness above thy fellows." The first sentence I did not apply to myself; but being then, as I supposed, a man restored to himself, it was easy to feel that I had been anointed with the oil of gladness above my fellows. "Oil of gladness" is, in truth, an apt phrase wherewith to describe elation.

The last two verses of the psalm corroborated the messages

found in the preceding verses: "I will make thy name to be remembered in all generations:"—thus the minister. "Therefore shall the people praise thee for ever and ever," was the response I read. That spelled immortal fame for me, but only on condition that I should carry to a successful conclusion the mission of reform—an obligation placed upon me by God when He restored my reason.

When I set out upon a career of reform, I was impelled to do so by motives in part like those which seem to have possessed Don Quixote when he set forth, as Cervantes says, with the intention "of righting every kind of wrong, and exposing himself to peril and danger, from which in the issue he would obtain eternal renown and fame." In likening myself to Cervantes' mad hero my purpose is quite other than to push myself within the charmed circle of the chivalrous. What I wish to do is to make plain that a man abnormally elated may be swayed irresistibly by his best instincts, and that while under the spell of an exaltation, idealistic in degree, he may not only be willing, but eager to assume risks and endure hardships which under normal conditions he would assume reluctantly, if at all. In justice to myself, however, I may remark that my plans for reform have never assumed quixotic, and, therefore, impracticable, proportions. At no time have I gone a-tilting at windmills. A pen rather than a lance has been my weapon of offence and defence; for with its point I have felt sure that I should one day prick the civic conscience into a compassionate activity, and thus bring into a neglected field earnest men and women who should act as champions for those afflicted thousands least able to fight for themselves.

◈XIV◈

After being without relatives and friends for over two years I naturally lost no time in trying again to get in touch with them; though I did heed my conservator's request that I first give him two or three days in which to acquaint intimates with the new turn my affairs had taken.

During the latter part of that first week I wrote many letters, so many, indeed, that I soon exhausted a liberal supply of stationery. This had been placed at my disposal at the suggestion of my conservator, who had wisely arranged that I should have whatever I wanted, if expedient. It was now at my own suggestion that the supervisor gave me large sheets of manila wrapping paper. These I proceeded to cut into strips a foot wide. One such strip, four feet long, would suffice for a mere *billet-doux*; but a real letter usually required several such strips pasted together. More than once letters twenty or thirty feet long were written; and on one occasion the accumulation of two or three days of excessive productivity, when spread upon the floor, reached from one end of the corridor to the other— a distance of about one hundred feet. My hourly output was something like twelve feet, with an average of one hundred and fifty words to the foot. Under the pressure of elation one takes pride in doing everything in record time. Despite my speed my letters were not incoherent. They were simply digressive, which was to be expected, as elation befogs one's "goal idea." Though these epistolary monstrosities were launched, few reached those to whom they were addressed; for my conservator had wisely ordered that my literary output be sent in bulk to him. His action was exasperating, but later I realized that he had done me a great favor when he interposed his judgment between my red-hot mentality and the cool minds of the workaday world. Yet this interference with what I deemed my rights proved to be the first step in the general overruling of them by tactless attendants and, in particular, by a certain assistant physician.

I had always shown a strong inclination to superintend. In consequence, in my elated condition it was but natural that I should have an excess of executive impulses. In order to decrease this executive pressure I proceeded to assume entire charge of that portion of the hospital in which I happened at the moment to be confined. What I eventually issued as imperative orders were often presented at first as polite suggestions. But, if my suggestions were not accorded a respectful hearing, and my demands acted upon at once, I invariably supplemented them with vituperative ultimatums. These were double-edged, and involved me in trouble quite as often as they gained the ends I sought.

The assistant physician in charge of my case, realizing that he could not grant all of my requests, unwisely decided to deny most of them. Had he been tactful, he could have taken the same stand without arousing my animosity. As it was, he treated me with a contemptuous sort of indifference which finally developed into spite, and led to much trouble for us both. During the two wild months that followed, the superintendent and the steward could induce me to do almost anything by simply requesting it. If two men out of three could control me easily during such a period of mental excitement, is it not reasonable to suppose that the third man, the assistant physician, could likewise have controlled me had he treated me with consideration? It was his undisguised superciliousness that gave birth to my contempt for him. In a letter written during my second week of elation, I expressed the opinion that he and I should get along well together. But that was before I had become troublesome enough to try the man's patience. Nevertheless, it indicates that he could have saved himself hours of time and subsequent worry, had he met my friendly advances in the proper spirit, for it is the quality of heart quite as much as the quantity of mind that cures or makes happy the insane.

The literary impulse took such a hold on me that, when I first sat down to compose a letter, I bluntly refused to stop writing and go to bed when the attendant ordered me to do so. For over one year this man had seen me mute and meek, and the sudden and startling change from passive obedience to uncompromising independence naturally puzzled him. He threatened to drag me to my room, but strangely decided not to do so. After half an hour's futile coaxing, during which time an unwonted supply of blood was drawn to his brain, that surprised organ proved its gratitude by giving birth to a timely and sensible idea. With an unaccustomed resourcefulness, by cutting off the supply of light at the electric switch, he put the entire ward in darkness. Secretly I admired the stratagem, but my words on that occasion probably conveyed no idea of the approbation that lurked within me.

I then went to bed, but not to sleep. The ecstasy of elation made each conscious hour one of rapturous happiness, and my memory knows no day of brighter sunlight than those nights. The floodgates of thought were wide open. So jealous of each other were the thoughts they they seemed to stumble over one another in their mad rush to present themselves to my re-enthroned ego.

I naturally craved companionship, but there were not many patients whom I cared to talk with. I did, however, greatly desire to engage the assistant physician in conversation, as he was a man of some education and familiar with the history of my case. But this man, who had tried to induce me to speak when delusions had tied my tongue, now, when I was at last willing to talk, would scarcely condescend to listen; and what seemed to me his studied and ill-disguised avoidance only served to whet my desire to detain him whenever possible.

It was about the second week that my reformative turn of mind became acute. The ward in which I was confined was well furnished and as homelike as such a place could be, though in justice to my own home I must observe that the resemblance was not great. About the so-called violent ward I had far less favorable ideas. Though I had not been subjected to physical abuse during the first fourteen months of my stay here, I had seen unnecessary and often brutal force used by the attendants in managing several so-called violent patients, who, upon their arrival, had been placed in the ward where I was. I had also heard convincing rumors of rough treatment of irresponsible patients in the violent ward.

At once I determined to conduct a thorough investigation of the institution. In order that I might have proof that my intended action was deliberate, my first move was to tell one or two fellow-patients that I should soon transgress some rule in such a way as to necessitate my removal to the violent ward. At first I thought of breaking a few panes of glass; but my purpose was accomplished in another way—and, indeed, sooner than I had anticipated. My conservator, in my presence, had told the assistant physician that the doctors could permit me to telephone him whenever they should see fit. It was rather with the wish to test the unfriendly physician than to satisfy any desire to speak with my conservator that one morning I asked permission to call up the latter. That very morning I had received a letter from him. This the doctor knew, for I showed him the letter—but not its contents. It was on the letter that I based my demand, though in it my brother did not even intimate that he wished to speak to me. The doctor, however, had no way of knowing that my statement was not true. To deny my request was simply one of his ill-advised whims, and his refusal was given with customary curtness and contempt. I met his refusal in kind, and presented him with a trenchant critique of his character.

He said, "Unless you stop talking in that way I shall have you transferred to the Fourth Ward." (This was the violent ward.)

"Put me where you please," was my reply. "I'll put you in the gutter before I get through with you."

With that the doctor made good his threat, and the attendant escorted me to the violent ward—a willing, in fact, eager prisoner.

The ward in which I was now placed (September 13th, 1902) was furnished in the plainest manner. The floors were of hard wood and the walls were bare. Except when at meals or out of doors taking their accustomed exercise, the patients usually lounged about in one large room, in which heavy benches were used, it being thought that in the hands of violent patients, chairs might become a menace to others. In the dining room, however, there were chairs of a substantial type, for patients seldom run amuck at meal time. Nevertheless, one of these dining-room chairs soon acquired a history.

As my banishment had come on short notice, I had failed to provide myself with many things I now desired. My first request was that I be supplied with stationery. The attendants, acting no doubt on the doctor's orders, refused to grant my request; nor would they give me a lead pencil—which, luckily, I did not need, for I happened to have one. Despite their refusal I managed to get some scraps of paper, on which I was soon busily engaged in writing notes to those in authority. Some of these (as I learned later) were delivered, but no attention was paid to them. No doctor came near me until evening, when the one who had banished me made his regular round of inspection.

When he appeared, the interrupted conversation of the morning was resumed—that is, by me—and in a similar vein. I again asked leave to telephone my conservator. The doctor again refused, and, of course, again I told him what I thought of him.

My imprisonment pleased me. I was where I most wished to be, and I busied myself investigating conditions and making mental notes. As the assistant physician could grant favors to the attendants, and had authority to discharge them, they did his bidding and continued to refuse most of my requests. In spite of their unfriendly attitude, however, I did manage to persuade the supervisor, a kindly man, well along in years, to deliver a note to the steward. In it I asked him to come at once, as I wished to talk with him. The steward, whom I looked upon as a friend, returned no answer and made no visit. I supposed he, too, had purposely ignored me. As I learned afterwards, both he and the superintendent were absent, else perhaps I should have been treated in a less high-handed manner by the assistant physician, who was not absent.

The next morning, after a renewal of my request and a repeated refusal, I asked the doctor to send me the "Book of Psalms" which I had left in my former room. With this request he complied, believing, perhaps, that some religion would at least do me no harm. I probably read my favorite psalm, the 45th; but most of my time I spent writing, on the flyleaves, psalms of my own. And if the value of a psalm is to be measured by the intensity of feeling portrayed, my compositions of that day rightly belonged beside the writings of David. My psalms were indited to those in authority at the hospital, and later in the day the supervisor—who proved himself a friend on many occasions—took the book to headquarters.

The assistant physician, who had mistaken my malevolent tongue for a violent mind, had placed me in exile which precluded my attending the service which was held in the chapel that Sunday afternoon. Time which might better have been spent in church I therefore spent in perfecting a somewhat ingenious scheme for getting in touch with the steward. That evening, when the doctor again appeared, I approached him in a friendly way and politely repeated my request. He again refused to grant it. With an air of resignation I said, "Well, as it seems useless to argue the point with you I should like, with your kind permission, to kick a hole in your damned old building and to-morrow present myself to the steward in his office."

"Kick away!" he said with a sneer. He then entered an adjoining ward, where he remained for about ten minutes.

If you will draw in your mind, or on paper, a letter "L," and let the vertical part represent a room forty feet in length, and the horizontal part one of twenty, and if you will then picture me as standing in a doorway at the intersection of these two lines—the door to the dining room—and the doctor behind another door at the top of the perpendicular, forty feet away, you will have represented graphically the opposing armies just prior to the first real assault in what proved to be a siege of seven weeks.

The moment the doctor re-entered the ward, as he had to do to return to the office, I disappeared through my door—into the dining room. I then walked the length of that room and picked up one of the heavy wooden chairs, selected for my purpose while the doctor and his tame charges were at church. Using the chair as a battering-ram, without malice—joy being in my heart—I deliberately thrust two of its legs through an upper and a lower pane of a four-paned plate glass window. The only miscalculation I made was in failing to place myself directly in front of that window, and at a proper distance, so that I might have broken every one of the four panes. This was a source of regret to me, for I was always loath to leave a well-thought-out piece of work unfinished.

The crash of shattered and falling glass startled every one

but me. Especially did it frighten one patient who happened to be in the dining room at the time. He fled. The doctor and the attendant who were in the adjoining room could not see me, or know what the trouble was; but they lost no time in finding out. Like the proverbial cold-blooded murderer who stands over his victim, weapon in hand, calmly awaiting arrest, I stood my ground, and, with a fair degree of composure, awaited the on-rush of the doctor and attendant. They soon had me in hand. Each taking an arm, they marched me to my room. This took not more than half a minute, but the time was not so short as to prevent my delivering myself of one more thumb-nail charac-terization of the doctor. My inability to recall that delineation, verbatim, entails no loss on literature. But one remark made as the doctor seized hold of me was apt, though not impromptu. "Well, doctor," I said, "knowing you to be a truthful man, I just took you at your word."

Senseless as this act appears it was the result of logical think-ing. The steward had entire charge of the building and ordered all necessary repairs. It was he whom I desired above all others to see, and I reasoned that the breaking of several dollars' worth of plate glass (for which later, to my surprise, I had to pay) would compel his attention on grounds of economy, if not those of the friendly interest which I now believed he had abandoned. Early the next morning, as I had hoped, the steward appeared. He approached me in a friendly way (as had been his wont) and I met him in a like manner. "I wish you would leave a little bit of the building," he said good naturedly.

"I will leave it all, and gladly, if you will pay some attention to my messages," was my rejoinder.

"Had I not been out of town," he replied, " I would have come to see you sooner." And this honest explanation I accepted.

I made known to the steward the assistant physician's be-havior in balking my desire to telephone my conservator. He agreed to place the matter before the superintendent, who had that morning returned. As proof of gratitude, I promised to suspend hostilities until I had had a talk with the superintendent. I made it quite plain, however, that should he fail to keep his word, I would further facilitate the ventilation of the violent ward. My faith in mankind was not yet wholly restored.

ᴂXVᴐ

A few hours later, without having witnessed anything of particular significance, except as it befell myself, I was transferred to my old ward. The superintendent, who had ordered this rehabilitation, soon appeared, and he and I had a satisfactory talk. He gave me to understand that he himself would in future look after my case, as he realized that his assistant lacked the requisite tact and judgment to cope with one of my temperament—and with that, my desire to telephone my conservator vanished.

Now no physician would like to have his wings clipped by a patient, even indirectly, and without doubt the man's pride was piqued as his incompetence was thus made plain. Thereafter, when he passed through the ward, he and I had frequent tilts. Not only did I lose no opportunity to belittle him in the presence of attendants and patients, but I even created such opportunities; so that before long he tried to avoid me whenever possible. But it seldom was possible. One of my chief amusements consisted in what were really one-sided interviews with him. Occasionally he was so unwise as to stand his ground for several minutes, and his arguments on such occasions served only to keep my temper at a vituperative heat. If there were any epithets which I failed to apply to him during the succeeding weeks of my association with him, they must have been coined since. The uncanny admixture of sanity displayed by me, despite my insane condition, was something this doctor could not comprehend. Remarks of mine, which he should have discounted or ignored, rankled as the insults of a sane and free man would have done. And his blunt and indiscriminate refusal of most of my requests prolonged my period of mental excitement.

After my return to my old ward I remained there for a period of three weeks. At that time I was a very self-centred individual. My large and varied assortment of delusions of grandeur made everything seem possible. There were few problems I hesitated to attack. With sufficient provocation I even attacked attendants—problems in themselves; but such fights as I subsequently engaged in were fights either for my own rights or the rights of others. Though for a while I got along fairly well with the attendants and as well as could be expected with the assistant physician, it soon became evident that these men felt that to know me more was to love me less. Owing to their lack of capacity for the work required of them, I was able to cause them endless annoyance. Many times a day I would tell the attendants what to do and what not to do, and tell them what I should do if my requests, suggestions, or orders were not immediately complied with. For over one year they had seen me in a passive, almost speechless condition, and they were, therefore, unable to understand my unwonted aggressions. The threat that I would chastise them for any disobedience of my orders they looked upon as a huge joke. So it was, until one day I incontinently cracked that joke against the head of one of them.

It began in this wise: Early in October there was placed in the ward a man whose abnormality for the most part consisted of an inordinate thirst for liquor. He was over fifty years of age, well educated, traveled, refined and of an artistic temperament. Congenial companions were scarce where I was, and he and I were soon drawn together in friendship. This man had been trapped into the institution by the subterfuge of relatives. As is common in such cases, many "white" lies had been resorted to in order to save trouble for all concerned—that is, all except the patient. To be taken without notice from one's home and by a deceitful, though under the circumstances perhaps justifiable strategy, placed in a ward with fifteen other men, all exhibiting insanity in varying degrees, is as heartbreaking an ordeal as one can well imagine. Yet such was this man's experience. A free man one day, he found himself deprived of his liberty the next, and branded with what he considered an unbearable disgrace.

Mr. Blank (as I shall call him) was completely unnerved. As he was a stranger in what I well knew was a strange world, I took him under my protecting and commodious wing. I did all I could to cheer him up, and tried to secure for him that consideration which to me seemed indispensable to his well-being. Patients in his condition had never been forced, when taking their exercise, to walk about the grounds with the other patients. At no time during the preceding fourteen months had I seen a newly committed patient forced to exercise against his will. One who objected was invariably left in the ward, or his refusal was reported to the doctor before further action was taken. No sane person need stretch his imagination in order to realize how humiliating it would be for this man to walk with a crowd which greatly resembled a "chain gang." Two by two, under guard, these hostages of misfortune get the only long walks their restricted liberty allows them. After the one or two occasions when this man did walk with the gang, I was impressed with the not wholly unreasonable thought that the physical exercise in no way compensated for the mental distress which the sense of humiliation and disgrace caused him to suffer. It was delightfully easy for me to interfere on his behalf; and when he came to my room, wrought up over the prospect of another such humiliation and weeping bitterly, I assured him that he should take his exercise that day when I did. My first move to accomplish the desired result was to approach, in a friendly way, the attendant in charge, and ask him to permit my new friend to walk about the grounds with me when next I went. He said he would do nothing of the kind—that he intended to take this man when he took the others. I said, "For over a year I have been in this ward and so have you, and I have never yet seen a man in Mr. Blank's condition forced to go out of doors."

"It makes no difference whether you have or not," said the attendant, "he's going."

"Will you ask the doctor whether Mr. Blank can or cannot walk about the grounds with my special attendant when I go?"

"No, I won't. Furthermore, it's none of your business."

"If you resort to physical force and attempt to take Mr. Blank with the other patients, you'll wish you hadn't," I said, as I walked away.

At this threat the fellow scornfully laughed. To him it meant nothing. He believed I could fight only with my tongue, and I confess that I myself was in doubt as to my power of fighting otherwise.

Returning to my room, where Mr. Blank was in waiting, I supported his drooping courage and again assured him that he should be spared the dreaded ordeal. I ordered him to go to a certain room at the farther end of the hall and there await developments—so that, should there be a fight, the line of battle might be a long one. He obeyed. In a minute or two the attendant was headed for that room. I followed closely at his heels, still threatening to attack him if he dared so much as lay a finger on my friend. Though I was not then aware of it, I was followed by another patient, a man who, though a mental case, had his lucid intervals and always a loyal heart. He seemed to realize that trouble was brewing and that very likely I should need help. Once in the room, the war of words was renewed, my sensitive and unnerved friend standing by and anxiously looking on.

"I warn you once more," I said, "if you touch Mr. Blank, I'll punch you so hard you'll wish you hadn't." The attendant's answer was an immediate attempt to eject Mr. Blank from the room by force. Nothing could be more automatic than my action at that time; indeed, to this day I do not remember performing the act itself. What I remember is the determination to perform it and the subsequent evidence of its having been performed. At all events I had already made up my mind to do a certain thing if the attendant did a certain thing. He did the one and I did the other. Almost before he had touched Mr. Blank's person, my right fist struck him with great force in, on, or about the left eye. It was then that I became the object of the attendant's attention—but not his undivided attention—for as he was choking me, my unsuspected ally stepped up and paid the attendant a sincere compliment by likewise choking him. In the scuffle I was forced to the floor. The attendant had a grip upon my throat. My wardmate had a double grip upon the attendant's throat. Thus was formed a chain with a weak, if not a missing, link in the middle. Picture, if you will, an insane man being choked by a supposedly sane one, and he in turn being choked by a temporarily sane insane friend of the assaulted one, and you will have Nemesis as nearly in a nutshell as any mere rhetorician has yet been able to put her.

That I was well choked is proved by the fact that my throat bore the crescent-shaped mark of my assailant's thumb nail. And I am inclined to believe that my rescuer, who was a very powerful man, made a decided impression on my assailant's throat. Had not the superintendent opportunely appeared at that moment, the man might soon have lapsed into unconsciousness, for I am sure my ally would never have released him until he had released me. The moment the attendant with his one good eye caught sight of the superintendent the scrimmage ended. This was but natural, for it is against the code of honor generally obtaining among attendants, that one should so far forget himself as to abuse patients in the presence of sane and competent witnesses.

The choking which I had just received served only to limber my vocal cords. I told the doctor all about the preliminary verbal skirmish and the needlessness of the fight. The superintendent had graduated at Yale over fifty years prior to my own graduation, and because of this common interest and his consummate tact we got along well together. But his friendly interest did not keep him from speaking his mind upon occasion, as his words at this time proved. "You don't know," he said, "how it grieves me to see you—a Yale man—act so like a rowdy."

"If fighting for the rights of a much older man, unable to protect his own interests, is the act of a rowdy, I'm quite willing to be thought one," was my reply.

Need I add that the attendant did not take Mr. Blank for a walk that morning? Not, so far as I know, was the latter ever forced again to take his exercise against his will.

⁓XVI⁓

The superintendent now realized that I was altogether too energetic a humanitarian to remain in the ward with so many other patients. My actions had a demoralizing effect upon them; so I was forthwith transferred to a private room, one of two situated in a small one-story annex. These new quarters were rather attractive, not unlike a bachelor apartment.

As there was no one here with whom I could interfere I got along without making any disturbance—that is, so long as I had a certain special attendant, a man suited to my temperament. He who was now placed over me understood human nature. He never resorted to force if argument failed to move me; and trifling transgressions, which would have led to a fight had he behaved like a typical attendant, he either ignored or privately reported to the doctor. For the whole period of my intense excitement there were certain persons who could control me, and certain others whose presence threw me into a state bordering on rage, and frequently into passions which led to distressing results.

Unfortunately for me, my good attendant soon left the institution to accept a more attractive business offer. He left without even a good-bye to me. Nothing proves more conclusively how important to me would have been his retention than this abrupt leave-taking which the doctor had evidently ordered, thinking perhaps that the prospect of such a change would excite me.

However, I caused no trouble when the substitution was made, though I did dislike having placed over me a man with whom I had previously had misunderstandings. He was about my own age and it was by no means so easy to take orders from him as it had been to obey his predecessor, who was considerably older than myself. Then, too, this younger attendant disliked me because of the many disagreeable things I had said to him while we were together in a general ward. He weighed about one hundred and ninety pounds to my one hundred and thirty, and had evidently been selected to attend me because of his great strength. A choice based on mental rather than physical considerations would have been wiser. The superintendent, because of his advanced age and ill health, had been obliged again to place my case in the hands of the assistant physician, and the latter gave this new attendant certain orders. What I was to be permitted to do, and what not, was carefully specified. These orders, many of them unreasonable, were carried out to the letter. For this I cannot justly blame the attendant. The doctor had deprived him of the right to exercise what judgment he had.

At this period I required but little sleep. I usually spent part of the night drawing; for it was in September, 1902, while I was at the height of my wave of self-centred confidence, that I decided that I was destined to become a writer of books—or at least of one book; and now I thought I might as well be an artist, too, and illustrate my own works. In school I had never cared for drawing; nor at college either. But now my awakened artistic impulse was irresistible. My first self-imposed lesson was a free-hand copy of an illustration on a cover of *Life*. Considering the circumstances, that first drawing was creditable, though I cannot now prove the assertion; for inconsiderate attendants destroyed it, with many more of my drawings and manuscripts. From the very moment I completed that first drawing, honors were divided between my literary and artistic impulses; and a letter which, in due time, I felt impelled to write to the Governor of the State, incorporated art with literature. I wrote and read several hours a day and I spent as many more in drawing. But the assistant physician, instead of making it easy for me to rid myself of an excess of energy along literary and artistic lines, balked me at every turn, and seemed to delight in displaying as little interest as possible in my newly awakened ambitions. When everything should have been done to calm my abnormally active mind, a studied indifference and failure to protect my interests kept me in a state of exasperation.

But circumstances now arose which brought about the untimely stifling—I might better say strangulation—of my artistic impulses. The doctors were led—unwisely, I believe—to decide that absolute seclusion was the only thing that would calm my over-active brain. In consequence, all writing and drawing materials and all books were taken from me. And from October 18th until the first of the following January, except for one fortnight, I was confined in one or another small, barred room, hardly better than a cell in a prison and in some instances far worse.

A corn cob was the determining factor at this crisis. Seeing in myself an embryonic Raphael, I had a habit of preserving all kinds of odds and ends as souvenirs of my development. These, I believed, sanctified by my Midas-like touch, would one day be of great value. If the public can tolerate, as it does, thousands of souvenir hunters, surely one with a sick mind should be indulged in the whim for collecting such souvenirs as come within his reach. Among the odds and ends that I had gathered were several corn cobs. These I intended to gild and some day make useful by attaching to them small thermometers. But on the morning of October 18th, the young man in charge of me, finding the corn cobs, forthwith informed me that he would throw them away. I as promptly informed him that any such action on his part would lead to a fight. And so it did.

When this fight began, there were two attendants at hand. I fought them both to a standstill, and told them I should continue to fight until the assistant physician came to the ward. Thereupon, my special attendant, realizing that I meant what I said, held me while the other went for assistance. He soon returned, not with the assistant physician, but with a third attendant, and the fight was renewed. The one who had acted as messenger, being of finer fibre than the other two, stood at a safe distance. It was, of course, against the rules of the institution for an attendant to strike a patient, and, as I was sane enough to report with a fair chance of belief any forbidden blows, each captor had to content himself with holding me by an arm and attempting to choke me into submission. However, I was able to prevent them from getting a good grip on my throat, and for almost ten minutes I continued to fight, telling them all the time that I would not stop until a doctor should come. An assistant physician, but not the one in charge of my case, finally appeared. He gave orders that I be placed in the violent ward, which adjoined the private apartment I was then occupying, and no time was lost in locking me in a small room in that ward.

Friends have said to me: "Well, what is to be done when a patient runs amuck?" The best answer I can make is: "Do nothing to make him run amuck." Psychiatrists have since told me that had I had an attendant with the wisdom and ability to humor me and permit me to keep my priceless corn cobs, the fight in question, and the worse events that followed, would probably not have occurred—not that day, nor ever, had I at all times been properly treated by those in charge of me.

So again I found myself in the violent ward—but this time not because of any desire to investigate it. Art and literature being now more engrossing than my plans for reform, I became, in truth, an unwilling occupant of a room and ward devoid of even a suggestion of the æsthetic. The room itself was clean, and under other circumstances might have been cheerful. It was twelve feet long, seven feet wide, and twelve high. A cluster of incandescent lights, enclosed in a semi-spherical glass globe, was attached to the ceiling. The walls were bare and plainly wainscotted, and one large window, barred outside, gave light. At one side of the door was an opening a foot square with a door of its own which could be unlocked only from without, and through which food could be passed to a supposedly dangerous patient. Aside from a single bed, the legs of which were screwed to the floor, the room had no furniture.

The attendant, before locking me in, searched me and took from me several lead pencils; but the stub of one escaped his vigilance. Naturally, to be taken from a handsomely furnished apartment and thrust into such a bare and unattractive room as this caused my already heated blood to approach the boiling point. Consequently, my first act was to send a note to the physician who regularly had charge of my case, requesting him to visit me as soon as he should arrive, and I have every reason to believe that the note was delivered. Whether or not this was so, a report of the morning's fight and my transfer must have reached him by some of several witnesses. While waiting for an answer, I busied myself writing, and as I had no stationery I wrote on the walls. Beginning as high as I could reach, I wrote in columns, each about three feet wide. Soon the pencil became dull. But dull pencils are easily sharpened on the whetstone of wit. Stifling acquired traits I permitted myself to revert momentarily to a primitive expedient. I gnawed the wood quite from the pencil, leaving only the graphite core. With a bit of graphite a hand guided by the unerring insolence of elation may artistically damn all men and things. That I am inclined to believe I did; and I question whether Raphael or Michael Angelo—upon whom I then looked as mere predecessors—ever put more feeling per square foot into their mural masterpieces. Every little while, as if to punctuate my composition, and in an endeavor to get attention, I viciously kicked the door.

This first fight of the day occurred about 8 A.M. For the three hours following I was left to thrash about the room and work myself into a frenzy. I made up my mind to compel attention. A month earlier, shattered glass had enabled me to accomplish a certain sane purpose. Again this day it served me. The opalescent half-globe on the ceiling seemed to be the most vulnerable point for attack. How to reach and smash it was the next question—and soon answered. Taking off my shoes, I threw one with great force at my glass target and succeeded in striking it a destructive blow.

The attendants charged upon my room. Their entrance was momentarily delayed by the door which stuck fast. I was standing near it, and when it gave way, its edge struck me on the forehead with force enough to have fractured my skull had it struck a weaker part. Once in the room, the two attendants threw me on the bed and one choked me so severely that I could feel my eyes starting from their sockets. The attendants then put the room in order; removed the glass—that is, all except one small and apparently innocent, but as the event proved well-nigh fatal, piece—took my shoes and again locked me in my room—not forgetting, however, to curse me well for making them work for their living.

When the assistant physician finally appeared, I met him with a blast of invective which, in view of the events which quickly followed, must have blown out whatever spark of kindly feeling toward me he may ever have had. I demanded that he permit me to send word to my conservator asking him to come at once and look after my interests, for I was being unfairly treated. I also demanded that he request the superintendent to visit me at once, as I intended to have nothing more to do with the assistant physicians or attendants who were neglecting and abusing me. He granted neither demand.

The bit of glass which the attendants had overlooked was about the size of my thumb nail. If I remember rightly, it was not a part of the broken globe. It was a piece that had probably been hidden by a former occupant, in a corner of the square opening at the side of the door. At all events, if the pen is the tongue of a ready writer, so may a piece of glass be, under given conditions. As the thought I had in mind seemed an immortal one I decided to etch, rather than write with fugitive graphite. On the topmost panel of the door, which a few minutes before had dealt me so vicious a blow, I scratched a seven-word sentiment—sincere, if not classic: "God bless our Home, which is Hell."

The violent exercise of the morning had given me a good appetite and I ate my dinner with relish, though with some difficulty, for the choking had lamed my throat. On serving this dinner, the attendants again left me to my own devices. The early part of the afternoon I spent in vain endeavors to summon them and induce them to take notes to the superintendent and his assistant. They continued to ignore me. By sundown the furious excitement of the morning had given place to what might be called a deliberative excitement, which, if anything, was more effective. It was but a few days earlier that I had discussed my case with the assistant physician and told him all about the suicidal impulse which had been so strong during my entire period of depression. I now reasoned that a seeming attempt at suicide, a "fake" suicide, would frighten the attendants into calling this doctor whose presence I now desired—and desired the more because of his studied indifference. No man that ever lived, loved life more than I did on that day, and the mock tragedy which I successfully staged about dusk was, I believe, as good a farce as was ever perpetrated. If I had any one ambition it was to live long enough to regain my freedom and put behind prison bars this doctor and his burly henchmen. To compel attention that was my object.

At this season the sun set by half-past five and supper was usually served about that time. So dark was my room then that objects in it could scarcely be discerned. About a quarter of an hour before the attendant was due to appear with my evening meal I made my preparations. That the stage setting might be in keeping with the plot, I tore up such papers as I had with me, and also destroyed other articles in the room—as one might do in a frenzy; and to complete the illusion of desperation, deliberately broke my watch. I then took off my suspenders, and tying one end to the head of the bedstead, made a noose of the other. At the crucial moment I placed my pillow on the floor beside the head of the bed and sat on it—for this was to be an easy death. I then bore just enough weight on the improvised noose to give all a plausible look. And a last lifelike (or rather death-like) touch I added by gurgling as in infancy's happy days.

No schoolboy ever enjoyed a prank more than I enjoyed this one. Soon I heard the step of the attendant, bringing my supper. When he opened the door, he had no idea that anything unusual was happening within. Coming as he did from a well-lighted room into one that was dark, it took him several seconds to grasp the situation—and then he failed really to take it in, for he at once supposed me to be in a semi-unconscious condition from strangulation. In a state of great excitement this brute of the morning called to his brute partner and I was soon released from what was nothing more than an amusing position, though they believed it one of torture or death. The vile curses with which they had addressed me in the morning were now silenced. They spoke kindly and expressed regret that I should have seen fit to resort to such an act. Their sympathy was as genuine as such men can feel, but a poor kind at best, for it was undoubtedly excited by the thought of what might be the consequences to them of their own neglect. While this unwonted stress of emotion threatened their peace of mind, I continued to play my part, pretending to be all but unconscious.

Shortly after my rescue from a very living death, the attendants picked me up and carried my limp body and laughing soul to an adjoining room, where I was tenderly placed upon a bed. I seemed gradually to revive.

"What did you do it for?" asked one.

"What's the use of living in a place like this, to be abused as I've been today?" I asked. "You and the doctor ignore me and all my requests. Even a cup of water between meals is denied me, and other requests which you have no right to refuse. Had I killed myself, both of you would have been discharged. And if my relatives and friends had ever found out how you had abused and neglected me, it is likely you would have been arrested and prosecuted."

Word had already been sent to the physician. He hurried to the ward, his almost breathless condition showing how my farce had been mistaken for real tragedy. The moment he entered I abandoned the part I had been playing.

"Now that I have you three brutes where I want you, I'll tell you a few things you don't know," I said. "You probably think I've just tried to kill myself. It was simply a ruse to make you give me some attention. When I make threats and tell you that my one object in life is to live long enough to regain my freedom and lay bare the abuses which abound in places like this, you simply laugh at me, don't you? But the fact is, that's my ambition, and if you knew anything at all, you'd know that abuse won't drive me to suicide. You can continue to abuse me and deprive me of my rights, and keep me in exile from relatives and friends, but the time will come when I'll make you sweat for all this. I'll put you in prison where you belong. Or if I fail to do that, I can at least bring about your discharge from this institution. What's more, I will."

The doctor and attendants took my threats with characteristic nonchalance. Such threats, often enough heard in such places, make little or no impression, for they are seldom made good. When I made these threats, I really wished to put these men in prison. Today I have no such desire, for were they not victims of the same vicious system of treatment to which I was subjected? In every institution where the discredited principles of "Restraint" are used or tolerated, the very atmosphere is brutalizing. Place a bludgeon in the hand of any man, with instructions to use it when necessary, and the gentler and more humane methods of persuasion will naturally be forgotten or deliberately abandoned.

Throughout my period of elation, especially the first months of it when I was doing the work of several normal men, I required an increased amount of fuel to generate the abnormal energy my activity demanded. I had a voracious appetite, and I insisted that the attendant give me the supper he was about to serve when he discovered me in the simulated throes of death. At first he refused, but finally relented and brought me a cup of tea and some buttered bread. Because of the severe choking administered earlier in the day it was with difficulty that I swallowed any food. I *had* to eat slowly. The attendant, however, ordered me to hurry, and threatened otherwise to take what little supper I had. I told him that I thought he would not —that I was entitled to my supper and intended to eat it with as much comfort as possible. This nettled him, and by a sudden and unexpected move he managed to take from me all but a crust of bread. Even that he tried to snatch. I resisted and the third fight of the day was on—and that within five minutes of the time the doctor had left the ward. I was seated on the bed. The attendant, true to his vicious instincts, grasped my throat and choked me with the full power of a hand accustomed to that unmanly work. His partner, in the meantime, had rendered me helpless by holding me flat on my back while the attacking party choked me into breathless submission. The first fight of the day was caused by a corn cob; this of the evening by a crust of bread.

Were I to close the record of events of that October day with an account of the assault just described, few, if any, would imagine that I had failed to mention all the abuse to which I was that day subjected. The fact is that not the half has been told. As the handling of me within the twenty-four hours typifies the worst, but, nevertheless, the not unusual treatment of patients in a like condition, I feel constrained to describe minutely the torture which was my portion that night.

There are several methods of restraint in use to this day in various institutions, chief among them "mechanical restraint" and so-called "chemical restraint." The former consists in the use of instruments of restraint, namely, strait-jackets or camisoles, muffs, straps, mittens, restraint of strong sheets, etc.—all of them, except on the rarest of occasions, instruments of neglect and torture. Chemical restraint (sometimes called medical restraint) consists in the use of temporarily paralyzing drugs—hyoscine being the popular "dose." By the use of such drugs a troublesome patient may be rendered unconscious and kept so for hours at a time. Indeed, very troublesome patients (especially when attendants are scarce) are not infrequently kept in a stupefied condition for days, or even for weeks—but only in institutions where the welfare of the patients is lightly regarded.

After the supper fight I was left alone in my room for about an hour. Then the assistant physician entered with three attendants, including the two who had figured in my farce. One carried a canvas contrivance known as a camisole. A camisole is a type of strait-jacket; and a very convenient type it is for those who resort to such methods of restraint, for it enables them to deny the use of strait-jackets at all. A strait-jacket, indeed, is not a camisole, just as electrocution is not hanging.

A camisole, or, as I prefer to stigmatize it, a strait-jacket, is really a tight-fitting coat of heavy canvas, reaching from neck to waist, constructed, however, in no ordinary pattern. There is not a button on it. The sleeves are closed at the ends, and the jacket, having no opening in front, is adjusted and tightly laced behind. To the end of each blind sleeve is attached a strong cord. The cord on the right sleeve is carried to the left of the body, and the cord on the left sleeve is carried to the right of the body. Both are then drawn tightly behind, thus bringing the arms of the victim into a folded position across his chest. These cords are then securely tied.

When I planned my ruse of the afternoon, I knew perfectly that I should soon find myself in a strait-jacket. The thought rather took my fancy, for I was resolved to know the inner workings of the violent ward.

The piece of glass with which I had that morning written the motto already quoted, I had appropriated for a purpose. Knowing that I should soon be put in the uncomfortable, but not necessarily intolerable embrace of a strait-jacket, my thought was that I might during the night, in some way or other, use this piece of glass to advantage—perhaps cut my way to a limited freedom. To make sure that I should retain possession of it, I placed it in my mouth and held it snugly against my cheek. Its presence there did not interfere with my speech; nor did it invite visual detection. But had I known as much about strait-jackets and their adjustment as I learned later, I should have resorted to no such futile expedient.

After many nights of torture, this jacket, at my urgent and repeated request, was finally adjusted in such manner that, had it been so adjusted at first, I need not have suffered any *torture* at all. This I knew at the time, for I had not failed to discuss the matter with a patient who on several occasions had been restrained in this same jacket.

On this occasion the element of personal spite entered into the assistant physician's treatment of me. The man's personality was apparently dual. His "Jekyll" personality was the one most in evidence, but it was the "Hyde" personality that seemed to control his actions when a crisis arose. It was "Doctor Jekyll" who approached my room that night, accompanied by the attendants. The moment he entered my room he became "Mr. Hyde." He was, indeed, no longer a doctor, or the semblance of one. His first move was to take the strait-jacket in his own hands and order me to stand. Knowing that those in authority really believed I had that day attempted to kill myself, I found no fault with their wish to put me in restraint; but I did object to having this done by Jekyll-Hyde. Though a strait-jacket should always be adjusted by the physician in charge, I knew that as a matter of fact the disagreeable duty was invariably assigned to the attendants. Consequently Jekyll-Hyde's eagerness to assume an obligation he usually shirked gave me the feeling that his motives were spiteful. For that reason I preferred to entrust myself to the uncertain mercies of a regular attendant; and I said so, but in vain. "If you will keep your mouth shut, I'll be able to do this job quicker," said Jekyll-Hyde.

"I'll shut my mouth as soon as you get out of this room and not before," I remarked. Nor did I. My abusive language was, of course, interlarded with the inevitable epithets. The more I talked, the more vindictive he became. He said nothing, but, unhappily for me, he expressed his pent-up feelings in something more effectual than words. After he had laced the jacket, and drawn my arms across my chest so snugly that I could not move them a fraction of an inch, I asked him to loosen the strait-jacket enough to enable me at least to take a full breath. I also requested him to give me a chance to adjust my fingers, which had been caught in an unnatural and uncomfortable position.

"If you will keep still a minute, I will," said Jekyll-Hyde. I obeyed, and willingly, too, for I did not care to suffer more than was necessary. Instead of loosening the appliance as agreed, this doctor, now livid with rage, drew the cords in such a way that I found myself more securely and cruelly held than before. This breach of faith threw me into a frenzy. Though it was because his continued presence served to increase my excitement that Jekyll-Hyde at last withdrew, it will be observed that he did not do so until he had satisfied an unmanly desire which an apparently lurking hatred had engendered. The attendants soon withdrew and locked me up for the night.

No incidents of my life have ever impressed themselves more indelibly on my memory than those of my first night in a straitjacket. Within one hour of the time I was placed in it I was suffering pain as intense as any I ever endured, and before the night had passed it had become almost unbearable. My right hand was so held that the tip of one of my fingers was all but cut by the nail of another, and soon knifelike pains began to shoot through my right arm as far as the shoulder. After four or five hours the excess of pain rendered me partially insensible to it. But for fifteen consecutive hours I remained in that instrument of torture; and not until the twelfth hour, about breakfast time the next morning, did the attendant so much as loosen a cord.

During the first seven or eight hours, excruciating pains racked not only my arms, but half of my body. Though I cried and moaned, in fact, screamed so loudly that the attendants must have heard me, little attention was paid to me—possibly because of orders from Mr. Hyde after he had again assumed the rôle of Doctor Jekyll. I even begged the attendants to loosen the jacket enough to ease me a little. This they refused to do, and they even seemed to enjoy being in a position to add their considerable mite to my torture.

Before midnight I really believed that I should be unable to endure the torture and retain my reason. A peculiar pricking sensation which I now felt in my brain, a sensation exactly like that of June, 1900, led me to believe that I might again be thrown out of touch with the world I had so lately regained. Realizing the awfulness of that fate, I redoubled my efforts to effect my rescue. Shortly after midnight I did succeed in gaining the attention of the night watch. Upon entering my room he found me flat upon the floor. I had fallen from the bed and perforce remained absolutely helpless where I lay. I could not so much as lift my head. This, however, was not the fault of the strait-jacket. It was because I could not control the muscles of my neck which that day had been so mauled. I could scarcely swallow the water the night watch was good enough to give me. He was not a bad sort; yet even he refused to let out the cords of the strait-jacket. As he seemed sympathetic, I can attribute his refusal to nothing but strict orders issued by the doctor.

It will be recalled that I placed a piece of glass in my mouth before the strait-jacket was adjusted. At midnight the glass was still there. After the refusal of the night watch, I said to him: "Then I want you to go to Dr. Jekyll" (I, of course, called him by his right name; but to do so now would be to prove myself as brutal as Mr. Hyde himself). "Tell him to come here at once and loosen this jacket. I can't endure the torture much longer. After fighting two years to regain my reason, I believe I'll lose it again. You have always treated me kindly. For God's sake, get the doctor."

"I can't leave the main building at this time," the night watch said. (Jekyll-Hyde lived in a house about one-eighth of a mile distant, but within the hospital grounds.)

"Then will you take a message to the assistant physician who stays here?" (A colleague of Jekyll-Hyde had apartments in the main building.)

"Tell him how I'm suffering. Ask him to please come here at once and ease this strait-jacket. If he doesn't, I'll be as crazy by morning as I ever was. Also tell him I'll kill myself unless he comes, and I can do it, too. I have a piece of glass in this room and I know just what I'll do with it."

The night watch was a good as his word. He afterwards told me that he had delivered my message. The doctor ignored it.

He did not come near me that night, nor the next day, nor did Jekyll-Hyde appear until his usual round of inspection about eleven o'clock the next morning.

"I understand that you have a piece of glass which you threatened to use for a suicidal purpose last night," he said, when he appeared.

"Yes, I have, and it's not your fault or the other doctor's that I am not dead. Had I gone mad, in my frenzy, I might have swallowed that glass."

"Where is it?" asked the doctor, incredulously.

As my strait-jacket rendered me armless, I presented the glass to Jekyll-Hyde on the tip of a tongue he had often heard, but never before seen.

~XVII~

After fifteen interminable hours the strait-jacket was removed. Whereas just prior to its putting on I had been in a vigorous enough condition to offer stout resistance when wantonly assaulted, now, on coming out of it, I was helpless. When my arms were released from their constricted position, the pain was intense. Every joint had been racked. I had no control over the fingers of either hand, and could not have dressed myself had I been promised my freedom for doing so.

For more than the following week I suffered as already described, though of course with gradually decreasing intensity as my racked body became accustomed to the unnatural positions it was forced to take. The first experience occurred on the night of October 18th, 1902. I was subjected to the same unfair, unnecessary, and unscientific ordeal for twenty-one consecutive nights and parts of the corresponding twenty-one days. On more than one occasion, indeed, the attendant placed me in the strait-jacket during the day for refusing to obey some trivial command. This, too, without an explicit order from the doctor in charge, though perhaps he acted under a general order.

During most of the time I was held also in seclusion in a padded cell. A padded cell is a vile hole. The side walls are padded as high as a man can reach, as is also the inside of the door. One of the worst features of such cells is the lack of ventilation, which deficiency of course aggravates their general unsanitary condition. The cell which I was forced to occupy was practically without heat, and as winter was coming on, I suffered intensely from the cold. Frequently it was so cold I could see my breath. Though my canvas jacket served to protect part of that body which it was at the same time racking, I was seldom comfortably warm; for, once uncovered, my arms being pinioned, I had no way of rearranging the blankets. What little sleep I managed to get I took lying on a hard mattress placed on the bare floor. The condition of the mattress I found in the cell was such that I objected to its further use, and the fact that another was supplied, at a time when few of my requests were being granted, proves its disgusting condition.

For this period of three weeks—from October 18th until November 8th, 1902, when I left this institution and was transferred to a state hospital—I was continuously either under lock and key (in the padded cell or some other room) or under the eye of an attendant. Over half the time I was in the snug, but cruel embrace of a strait-jacket—about three hundred hours in all.

While being subjected to this terrific abuse I was held in exile. I was cut off from all direct and all *honest* indirect communication with my legally appointed conservator—my own brother—and also with all other relatives and friends. I was even cut off from satisfactory communication with the superintendent. I saw him but twice, and then for so short a time that I was unable to give him any convincing idea of my plight. These interviews occurred on two Sundays that fell within my period of exile, for it was on Sunday that the superintendent usually made his weekly round of inspection.

What chance had I of successfully pleading my case, while my pulpit was a padded cell, and the congregation—with the exception of the superintendent—the very ones who had been abusing me? At such times my pent-up indignation poured itself forth in such a disconnected way that my protests were robbed of their right ring of truth. I was not incoherent in speech. I was simply voluble and digressive—a natural incident of elation. Such notes as I managed to write on scraps of paper were presumably confiscated by Jekyll-Hyde. At all events, it was not until some months later that the superintendent was informed of my treatment, when, at my request (though I was then elsewhere), the Governor of the State discussed the subject with him. How I brought about that discussion while still virtually a prisoner in another place will be narrated in due time. And not until several days after I had left this institution and had been placed in another, when for the first time in six weeks I saw my conservator, did *he* learn of the treatment to which I had been subjected. From his office in New Haven he had telephoned several times to the assistant physician and inquired about my condition. Though Jekyll-Hyde did tell him that I was highly excited and difficult to control, he did not even hint that I was being subjected to any unusual restraint. Doctor Jekyll deceived everyone, and—as things turned out—deceived himself; for had he realized then that I should one day be able to do what I have since done, his brutality would surely have been held in check by his discretion.

How helpless, how at the mercy of his keepers, a patient may be is further illustrated by the conduct of this same man. Once, during the third week of my nights in a strait-jacket, I refused to take certain medicine which an attendant offered me. For some time I had been regularly taking this innocuous concoction without protest; but I now decided that, as the attendant refused most of my requests, I should no longer comply with all of his. He did not argue the point with me. He simply reported my refusal to Doctor Jekyll. A few minutes later Doctor Jekyll —or rather Mr. Hyde—accompanied by three attendants, entered the padded cell. I was robed for the night—in a strait-jacket. Mr. Hyde held in his hand a rubber tube. An attendant stood near with the medicine. For over two years, the common threat had been made that the "tube" would be resorted to if I refused medicine or food. I had begun to look upon it as a myth; but its presence in the hands of an oppressor now convinced me of its reality. I saw that the doctor and his bravos meant business; and as I had already endured torture enough, I determined to make every concession this time and escape what seemed to be in store for me.

"What are you going to do with that?" I asked, eyeing the tube.

"The attendant says you refuse to take your medicine. We are going to make you take it."

"I'll take your old medicine," was my reply.

"You have had your chance."

"All right," I said. "Put that medicine into me in any way you think best. But the time will come when you'll wish you hadn't. When that time does come it won't be easy to prove that you had the right to force a patient to take medicine he had offered to take. I know something about the ethics of your profession. You have no right to do anything to a patient except what's good for him. You know that. All you are trying to do is to punish me, and I give you fair warning I'm going to camp on your trail till you are not only discharged from this institution, but expelled from the State Medical Society as well. You are a disgrace to your profession, and that society will attend to your case fast enough when certain members of it, who are friends of mine, hear about this. Furthermore, I shall report your conduct to the Governor of the State. He can take some action even if this is *not* a state institution. Now, damn you, do your worst!"

Coming from one in my condition, this was rather straight talk. The doctor was visibly disconcerted. Had he not feared to lose caste with the attendants who stood by, I think he would have given me another chance. But he had too much pride and too little manhood to recede from a false position already taken. I no longer resisted, even verbally, for I no longer wanted the doctor to desist. Though I did not anticipate the operation with pleasure, I was eager to take the man's measure. He and the attendants knew that I usually kept a trick or two even up the sleeve of a strait-jacket, so they took added precautions. I was flat on my back, with simply a mattress between me and the floor. One attendant held me. Another stood by with the medicine and with a funnel through which, as soon as Mr. Hyde should insert the tube in one of my nostrils, the dose was to be poured. The third attendant stood near as a reserve force. Though the insertion of the tube, when skillfully done, need not cause suffering, the operation as conducted by Mr. Hyde was painful. Try as he would, he was unable to insert the tube properly, though in no way did I attempt to balk him. His embarrassment seemed to rob his hand of whatever cunning it may have possessed. After what seemed ten minutes of bungling, though it was probably not half that, he gave up the attempt, but not until my nose had begun to bleed. He was plainly chagrined when he and his bravos retired. Intuitively I felt that they would soon return. That they did, armed with a new implement of war. This time the doctor inserted between my teeth a large wooden peg—to keep open a mouth which he usually wanted shut. He then forced down my throat a rubber tube, the attendant then adjusted the funnel, and the medicine, or rather liquid—for its medicinal properties were without effect upon me—was poured in.

As the scant reports sent to my conservator during these three weeks indicated that I was not improving as he had hoped, he made a special trip to the institution to investigate in person. On his arrival he was met by none other than Doctor Jekyll, who told him that I was in a highly excited condition, which, he intimated, would be aggravated by a personal interview. Now for a man to see his brother in such a plight as mine would be a distressing ordeal, and, though my conservator came within a few hundred feet of my prison cell, it naturally took but a suggestion to dissuade him from coming nearer. Doctor Jekyll did tell him that it had been found necessary to place me in "restraint" and "seclusion" (the professional euphemisms for "strait-jacket," "padded cell," etc.), but no hint was given that I had been roughly handled. Doctor Jekyll's politic dissuasion was no doubt inspired by the knowledge that if ever I got within speaking distance of my conservator, nothing could prevent my giving him a circumstantial account of my sufferings—which account would have been corroborated by the blackened eye I happened to have at the time. Indeed, in dealing with my conservator the assistant physician showed a degree of tact which, had it been directed toward myself, would have sufficed to keep me tolerably comfortable.

My conservator, though temporarily stayed, was not convinced. He felt that I was not improving where I was, and he wisely decided that the best course would be to have me transferred to a public institution—the State Hospital. A few days later the judge who had originally committed me ordered my transfer. Nothing was said to me about the proposed change until the moment of departure, and then I could scarcely believe my ears. In fact I did not believe my informant; for three weeks of abuse, together with my continued inability to get in touch with my conservator, had so shaken my reason that there was a partial recurrence of old delusions. I imagined myself on the way to the State Prison, a few miles distant; and not until the train had passed the prison station did I believe that I was really on my way to the State Hospital.

~XVIII~

The State Hospital in which I now found myself, the third institution to which I had been committed, though in many respects
above the average of such institutions, was typical. It com-
manded a wide view of a beautiful river and valley. This view
I was permitted to enjoy—at first. Those in charge of the institution which I had just left did not give my new custodians any
detailed account of my case. Their reticence was, I believe,
occasioned by chagrin rather than charity. Tamers of wild men
have as much pride as tamers of wild animals (but unfortunately less skill) and to admit defeat is a thing not to be thought
of. Though private institutions are prone to shift their troublesome cases to state institutions, there is too often a deplorable
lack of sympathy and co-operation between them, which in
this instance, however, proved fortunate for me.

From October 18th until the early afternoon of November
8th, at the private institution, I had been classed as a raving
maniac. The *name* I had brought upon myself by experimental
conduct; the *condition* had been aggravated and perpetuated by
the stupidity of those in authority over me. And it was the same
experimental conduct on my part, and stupidity on the part of
my new custodians, which gave rise, two weeks later, to a
similar situation. On Friday, November 7th, I was in a strait-
jacket. On November 9th and 10th I was apparently as tractable as any of the twenty-three hundred patients in the State

116

Hospital—conventionally clothed, mild mannered, and, seemingly, right minded. On the 9th, the day after my arrival, I attended a church service held at the hospital. My behavior was not other than that of the most pious worshipper in the land. The next evening, with most exemplary deportment, I attended one of the dances which are held every fortnight during the winter. Had I been a raving maniac, such activities would have led to a disturbance; for maniacs, of necessity, disregard the conventions of both pious and polite society. Yet, on either of these days, had I been in the private institution which I had recently left, I should have occupied a cell and worn a straitjacket.

The assistant superintendent, who received me upon my arrival, judged me by my behavior. He assigned me to one of two connecting wards—the best in the hospital—where about seventy patients led a fairly agreeable life. Though no official account of my case had accompanied my transfer, the attendant who had acted as escort and guard had already given an attendant at the State Hospital a brief account of my recent experiences. Yet when this report finally reached the ears of those in authority, they wisely decided not to transfer me to another ward so long as I caused no trouble where I was. Finding myself at last among friends, I lost no time in asking for writing and drawing materials, which had so rudely been taken from me three weeks earlier. My request was promptly granted. The doctors and attendants treated me kindly and I again began to enjoy life. My desire to write and draw had not abated. However, I did not devote my entire time to those pursuits, for there were plenty of congenial companions about. I found pleasure in talking—more pleasure by far than others did in listening. In fact I talked incessantly, and soon made known, in a general way, my scheme for reforming institutions, not only in my native State, but, of course, throughout the world, for my grandiose perspective made the earth look small. The attendants had to bear the brunt of my loquacity, and they soon grew weary. One of them, wishing to induce silence, ventured to remark that I was so "crazy" I could not possibly keep my mouth shut for even one minute. It was a challenge which aroused my fighting spirit.

"I'll show you that I can stop talking for a whole day," I said. He laughed, knowing that of all difficult tasks this which I had imposed upon myself was, for one in my condition, least likely of accomplishment. But I was as good as my boast. Until the same hour the next day I refused to speak to anyone. I did not even reply to civil questions; and though my silence was deliberate and good-natured, the assistant physician seemed to consider it of a contumacious variety, for he threatened to transfer me to a less desirable ward unless I should again begin to talk.

That day of self-imposed silence was about the longest I have ever lived, for I was under a word pressure sufficient to have filled a book. Any psychiatrist will admit that my performance was remarkable, and he will further agree that it was, at least, an indication of a high degree of self-control. Though I have no desire to prove that at this period I was not in an abnormal condition, I do wish to show that I had a degree of self-control that probably would have enabled me to remain in the best ward at this institution had I not been intent—abnormally intent, of course, and yet with a high degree of deliberation—upon a reformative investigation. The crest of my wave of elation had been reached early in October. It was now (November) that the curve representing my return to normality should have been continuous and diminishing. Instead, it was kept violently fluctuating—or at least its fluctuations were aggravated—by the impositions of those in charge of me, induced sometimes, I freely admit, by deliberate and purposeful transgressions of my own. My condition during my three weeks of exile just ended, had been, if anything, one of milder excitement than that which had obtained previously during the first seven weeks of my period of elation. And my condition during the two weeks I now remained in the best ward in the State Hospital was not different from my condition during the preceding three weeks of torture, or the succeeding three weeks of abuse and privation, except in so far as a difference was occasioned by the torture and privation themselves.

Though I had long intended to effect reforms in existing methods of treatment, my reckless desire to investigate violent wards did not possess me until I myself had experienced the torture of continued confinement in one such ward before coming to this state institution. It was simple to deduce that if one could suffer such abuses as I had while a patient in a private institution—nay, in two private institutions—brutality must exist in a state hospital also. Thus it was that I entered the State Hospital with a firm resolve to inspect personally every type of ward, good and bad.

But I was in no hurry to begin. My recent experiences had exhausted me, and I wished to regain strength before subjecting myself to another such ordeal. This desire to recuperate controlled my conduct for a while, but its influence gradually diminished as life became more and more monotonous. I soon found the good ward entirely too polite. I craved excitement— action. And I determined to get it regardless of consequences; though I am free to confess I should not have had the courage to proceed with my plan had I known what was in store for me.

About this time my conservator called to see me. Of course, I told him all about my cruel experiences at the private institution. My account surprised and distressed him. I also told him that I knew for a fact that similar conditions existed at the State Hospital, as I had heard convincing rumors to that effect. He urged me to behave myself and remain in the ward where I was, which ward, as I admitted, was all that one could desire— provided one had schooled himself to desire that sort of thing.

The fact that I was under lock and key and behind what were

virtually prison bars in no way gave me a sense of helplessness. I firmly believed that I should find it easy to effect my escape and reach home for the Thanksgiving Day celebration. And, furthermore, I knew that, should I reach home, I should not be denied my portion of the good things to eat before being returned to the hospital. Being under the spell of an intense desire to investigate the violent ward, I concluded that the time for action had come. I reasoned, too, that it would be easier and safer to escape from that ward—which was on a level with the ground—than from a ward three stories above it. The next thing I did was to inform the attendants (not to mention several of the patients) that within a day or two I should do something to cause my removal to it. They of course did not believe that I had any idea of deliberately inviting such a transfer. My very frankness disarmed them.

On the evening of November 21st, I went from room to room collecting all sorts of odds and ends belonging to other patients. These I secreted in my room. I had also collected a small library of books, magazines and newspapers. After securing all the booty I dared, I mingled with the other patients until the time came for going to bed. The attendants soon locked me in my junk shop and I spent the rest of the night setting it in disorder. My original plan had been to barricade the door during the night, and thus hold the doctors and attendants at bay until those in authority had accepted my ultimatum, which was to include a Thanksgiving visit at home. But before morning I had slightly altered my plan. My sleepless night of activity had made me ravenously hungry, and I decided that it would be wiser not only to fill my stomach, but to lay by other supplies of food before submitting to a siege. Accordingly I set things to rights and went about my business the next morning as usual. At breakfast I ate enough for two men, and put in my pockets bread enough to last for twenty-four hours at least. Then I returned to my room and at once barricaded the door. My barricade consisted of a wardrobe, several drawers which I had removed from the bureau and a number of books—among them "Paradise Lost" and the Bible. These, with conscious satisfaction, I placed in position as a keystone. Thus the floor space between the door and the opposite wall was completely filled. My roommate, a young fellow in the speechless condition in which I had been during my period of depression, was in the room with me. This was accidental. It was no part of my plan to hold him as a hostage, though I might finally have used him as a pawn in the negotiations, had my barricade resisted the impending attack longer than it did.

It was not long before the attendants realized that something was wrong. They came to my door and asked me to open it. I refused, and told them that to argue the point would be a waste of time. They tried to force an entrance. Failing in that, they reported to the assistant physician, who soon appeared. At first he parleyed with me. I good-naturedly, but emphatically, told him that I could not be talked out of the position I had taken; nor could I be taken out of it until I was ready to surrender, for my barricade was one that would surely hold. I also announced that I had carefully planned my line of action and knew what I was about. I complimented him on his hitherto tactful treatment of me, and grandiloquently—yet sincerely—thanked him for his many courtesies. I also expressed entire satisfaction with the past conduct of the attendants. In fact, on part of the institution I put my stamp of approval. "But," I said, "I know where there are wards in this hospital where helpless patients are brutally treated; and I intend to put a stop to these abuses at once. Not until the Governor of the State, the judge who committed me, and my conservator come to this door will I open it. When they arrive, we'll see whether or not patients are to be robbed of their rights and abused."

My speech was made through a screen transom over the door. For a few minutes the doctor continued his persuasive methods, but that he should even imagine that I would basely recede from my high and mighty position only irritated me the more.

"You can stand outside that door all day if you choose," I said. "I won't open it until the three men I have named appear. I have prepared for a siege; and I have enough food in this room to keep me going for a day anyway."

Realizing at last that no argument would move me, he set about forcing an entrance. First he tried to remove the transom by striking it with a stout stick. I gave blow for blow and the transom remained in place. A carpenter was then sent for, but before he could go about his work one of the attendants managed to open the door enough to thrust in his arm and shove aside my barricade. I did not realize what was being done until it was too late to interfere. The door once open, in rushed the doctor and four attendants. Without ceremony I was thrown upon the bed, with two or three of the attacking force on top of me. Again I was choked, this time by the doctor. The operation was a matter of only a moment. But before it was over I had the good fortune to deal the doctor a stinging blow on the jaw, for which (as he was about my own age and the odds were five to one) I have never felt called upon to apologize.

Once I was subdued, each of the four attendants attached himself to a leg or an arm and, under the direction and leadership of the doctor, I was carried bodily through two corridors, down two flights of stairs, and to the violent ward. My dramatic exit startled my fellow-patients, for so much action in so short a time is seldom seen in a quiet ward. And few patients placed in the violent ward are introduced with so impressive an array of camp-followers as I had that day.

All this to me was a huge joke, with a good purpose behind it. Though excited I was good-natured and, on the way to my new quarters, I said to the doctor: "Whether you believe it or not, it's a fact that I'm going to reform these institutions before I'm done. I raised this rumpus to make you transfer me to the violent ward. What I want you to do now is to show me the worst you've got."

"You needn't worry," the doctor said. "You'll get it."

He spoke the truth.

Even for a violent ward my entrance was spectacular—if not dramatic. The three attendants regularly in charge naturally jumped to the conclusion that, in me, a troublesome patient had been foisted upon them. They noted my arrival with an unpleasant curiosity, which in turn aroused *my* curiosity, for it took but a glance to convince me that my burly keepers were typical attendants of the brute-force type. Acting on the order of the doctor in charge, one of them stripped me of my outer garments; and, clad in nothing but underclothes, I was thrust into a cell.

Few, if any, prisons in this country contain worse holes than this cell proved to be. It was one of five, situated in a short corridor adjoining the main ward. It was about six feet wide by ten long and of a good height. A heavily screened and barred window admitted light and a negligible quantity of air, for the ventilation scarcely deserved the name. The walls and floor were bare, and there was no furniture. A patient confined here must lie on the floor with no substitute for a bed but one or two felt druggets. Sleeping under such conditions becomes tolerable after a time, but not until one has become accustomed to lying on a surface nearly as hard as a stone. Here (as well, indeed, as in other parts of the ward) for a period of three weeks I was again forced to breathe and rebreathe air so vitiated that even when I occupied a larger room in the same ward, doctors and attendants seldom entered without remarking its quality.

My first meal increased my distaste for my semi-sociological experiment. For over a month I was kept in a half-starved condition. At each meal, to be sure, I was given as much food as was served to other patients, but an average portion was not adequate to the needs of a patient as active as I was at this time.

Worst of all, winter was approaching and these, my first quarters, were without heat. As my olfactory nerves soon became uncommunicative, the breathing of foul air was not a hardship. On the other hand, to be famished the greater part of the time was a very conscious hardship. But to be half-frozen, day in and day out for a long period, was exquisite torture. Of all the suffering I endured, that occasioned by confinement in cold cells seems to have made the most lasting impression. Hunger is a local disturbance, but when one is cold, every nerve in the body registers its call for help. Long before reading a certain passage of De Quincey's I had decided that cold could cause greater suffering than hunger; consequently, it was with great satisfaction that I read the following sentences from his "Confessions": "O ancient women, daughters of toil and suffering, among all the hardships and bitter inheritances of flesh that ye are called upon to face, not one—not even hunger—seems in my eyes comparable to that of nightly cold. . . . A more killing curse there does not exist for man or woman than the bitter combat between the weariness that prompts sleep and the keen, searching cold that forces you from that first access of sleep to start up horror-stricken, and to seek warmth vainly in renewed exercise, though long since fainting under fatigue."

The hardness of the bed and the coldness of the room were not all that interfered with sleep. The short corridor in which I was placed was known as the "Bull Pen"—a phrase eschewed by the doctors. It was usually in an uproar, especially during the dark hours of the early morning. Patients in a state of excitement may sleep during the first hours of the night, but seldom all night; and even should one have the capacity to do so, his companions in durance would wake him with a shout or a song or a curse or the kicking of a door. A noisy and chaotic medley frequently continued without interruption for hours at a time. Noise, unearthly noise, was the poetic license allowed the occupants of these cells. I spent several days and nights in one or another of them, and I question whether I averaged more than two or three hours' sleep a night during that time. Seldom did the regular attendants pay any attention to the noise, though even they must at times have been disturbed by it. In fact the only person likely to attempt to stop it was the night watch, who, when he did enter a cell for that purpose, almost invariably kicked or choked a noisy patient into a state of temporary quiet. I noted this and scented trouble.

Drawing and writing materials having been again taken from me, I cast about for some new occupation. I found one in the problem of warmth. Though I gave repeated expression to the benumbed messages of my tortured nerves, the doctor refused to return my clothes. For a semblance of warmth I was forced to depend upon ordinary undergarments and an extraordinary imagination. The heavy felt druggets were about as plastic as blotting paper and I derived little comfort from them until I hit upon the idea of rending them into strips. These strips I would weave into a crude Rip Van Winkle kind of suit; and so intricate was the warp and woof that on several occasions an attendant had to cut me out of these sartorial improvisations. At first, until I acquired the destructive knack, the tearing of one drugget into strips was a task of four or five hours. But in time I became so proficient that I could completely destroy more than one of these six-by-eight-foot druggets in a single night. During the following weeks of my close confinement I destroyed at least twenty of them, each worth, as I found out later, about four dollars; and I confess I found a peculiar satisfaction in the destruction of property belonging to a State which had deprived me of all my effects except underclothes. But my destructiveness was due to a variety of causes. It was occasioned primarily by a "pressure of activity," for which the tearing of druggets served as a vent. I was in a state of mind aptly described in a letter written during my first month of elation, in which I said, "I'm as busy as a nest of ants."

Though the habit of tearing druggets was the outgrowth of an abnormal impulse, the habit itself lasted longer than it could have done had I not, for so long a time, been deprived of suitable clothes and been held a prisoner in cold cells. But another motive soon asserted itself. Being deprived of all the luxuries of life and most of the necessities, my mother wit, always conspiring with a wild imagination for something to occupy my time, led me at last to invade the field of invention. With appropriate contrariety, an unfamiliar and hitherto almost detested line of investigations now attracted me. Abstruse mathematical problems which had defied solution for centuries began to appear easy. To defy the State and its puny representatives had become mere child's play. So I forthwith decided to overcome no less a force than gravity itself.

My conquering imagination soon tricked me into believing that I could lift myself by my boot-straps—or rather that I could do so when my laboratory should ascertain footgear that lent itself to the experiment. But what of the strips of felt torn from the druggets? Why, these I used as the straps of my missing boots; and having no boots to stand in, I used my bed as boots. I reasoned that for my scientific purpose a man in bed was as favorably situated as a man in boots. Therefore, attaching a sufficient number of my felt strips to the head and foot of the bed (which happened not to be screwed to the floor), and in turn, attaching the free ends to the transom and window guard, I found the problem very simple. For I next joined these cloth cables in such a manner that by pulling downward I effected a readjustment of stress and strain, and my bed, *with me in it*, was soon dangling in space. My sensations at this momentous instant must have been much like those which thrilled Newton when he solved one of the riddles of the universe. Indeed, they must have been more intense, for Newton, knowing, had his doubts; I, not knowing, had no doubts at all. So epoch-making did this discovery appear to me that I noted the exact position of the bed so that a wondering posterity might ever afterward view and revere the exact spot on the earth's surface whence one of man's greatest thoughts had winged its way to immortality.

For weeks I believed I had uncovered a mechanical principle which would enable man to defy gravity. And I talked freely and confidently about it. That is, I proclaimed the impending results. The intermediate steps in the solution of my problem I ignored, for good reasons. A blind man may harness a horse. So long as the horse is harnessed, one need not know the office of each strap and buckle. Gravity was harnessed—that was all. Meanwhile I felt sure that another sublime moment of inspiration would intervene and clear the atmosphere, thus rendering flight of the body as easy as a flight of imagination.

✒ XX ✒

While my inventive operations were in progress, I was chafing under the unjust and certainly unscientific treatment to which I was being subjected. In spite of my close confinement in vile cells, for a period of over three weeks I was denied a bath. I do not regret this deprivation, for the attendants, who at the beginning were unfriendly, might have forced me to bathe in water which had first served for several other patients. Though such an unsanitary and disgusting practice was contrary to rules, it was often indulged in by the lazy brutes who controlled the ward.

I continued to object to the inadequate portions of food served me. On Thanksgiving Day (for I had not succeeded in escaping and joining in the celebration at home) an attendant, in the unaccustomed rôle of a ministering angel, brought me the usual turkey and cranberry dinner which, on two days a year, is provided by an intermittently generous State. Turkey being the *rara avis* of the imprisoned, it was but natural that I should desire to gratify a palate long insulted. I wished not only to satisfy my appetite, but to impress indelibly a memory which for months had not responded to so agreeable a stimulus. While lingering over the delights of this experience I forgot all about the ministering angel. But not for long. He soon returned. Observing that I had scarcely touched my feast, he said, "If you don't eat that dinner in a hurry, I'll take it from you."

"I don't see what difference it makes to you whether I eat it in a hurry or take my time about it," I said. "It's the best I've had in many a day, and I have a right to get as much pleasure out of it as I can."

"We'll see about that," he replied, and, snatching it away, he stalked out of the room, leaving me to satisfy my hunger on the memory of vanished luxuries. Thus did a feast become a fast.

Under this treatment I soon learned to be more noisy than my neighbors. I was never without a certain humor in contemplating not only my surroundings, but myself; and the demonstrations in which I began to indulge were partly in fun and partly by way of protest. In these outbursts I was assisted, and at times inspired, by a young man in the room next mine. He was about my own age and was enjoying the same phase of exuberance as myself. We talked and sang at all hours of the night. At the time we believed that the other patients enjoyed the spice which we added to the restricted variety of their lives, but later I learned that a majority of them looked upon us as the worst of nuisances.

We gave the doctors and attendants no rest—at least not intentionally. Whenever the assistant physician appeared, we upbraided him for the neglect which was then our portion. At one time or another we were banished to the Bull Pen for these indiscretions. And had there been a viler place of confinement still, our performances in the Bull Pen undoubtedly would have brought us to it. At last the doctor hit upon the expedient of transferring me to a room more remote from my inspiring, and, I may say, conspiring, companion. Talking to each other ceased to be the easy pastime it had been; so we gradually lapsed into a comparative silence which must have proved a boon to our ward-mates. The megaphonic Bull Pen, however, continued with irregularity, but annoying certainty to furnish its quota of noise.

On several occasions I concocted plans to escape, and not only that, but also to liberate others. That I did not make the attempt was the fault—or merit, perhaps—of a certain night watch, whose timidity, rather than sagacity, impelled him to refuse to unlock my door early one morning, although I gave him a plausible reason for the request. This night watch, I learned later, admitted that he feared to encounter me single-handed. And on this particular occasion well might he, for, during the night, I had woven a spider-web net in which I intended to enmesh him. Had I succeeded, there would have been a lively hour for him in the violent ward—had I failed, there would have been a lively hour for me. There were several comparatively sane patients (especially my elated neighbor) whose willing assistance I could have secured. Then the regular attendants could have been held prisoners in their own room, if, indeed, we had not in turn overpowered them and transferred them to the Bull Pen, where several victims of their abuse might have given them a deserved dose of their own medicine. This scheme of mine was a prank rather than a plot. I had an inordinate desire to prove that one *could* escape if he had a mind to do so. Later I boasted to the assistant physician of my unsuccessful attempt. This boast he evidently tucked away in his memory.

My punishment for harmless antics of this sort was prompt in coming. The attendants seemed to think their whole duty to their closely confined charges consisted in delivering three meals a day. Between meals he was a rash patient who interfered with their leisure. Now one of my greatest crosses was their continued refusal to give me a drink when I asked for it. Except at meal time, or on those rare occasions when I was permitted to go to the wash room, I had to get along as best I might with no water to drink, and that too at a time when I was in a fever of excitement. My polite requests were ignored; impolite demands were answered with threats and curses. And this war of requests, demands, threats, and curses continued until the night of the fourth day of my banishment. Then the attendants made good their threats of assault. That they had been trying to goad me into a fighting mood I well knew, and often accused them of their mean purpose. They brazenly admitted that they were simply waiting for a chance to "slug" me, and promised to punish me well as soon as I should give them a slight excuse for doing so.

On the night of November 25th, 1902, the head attendant and one of his assistants passed my door. They were returning from one of the dances which, at intervals during the winter, the management provides for the nurses and attendants. While they were within hearing, I asked for a drink of water. It was a carefully worded request. But they were in a hurry to get to bed, and refused me with curses. Then I replied in kind.

"If I come there I'll kill you," one of them said.

"Well, you won't get in if I can help it," I replied, as I braced my iron bedstead against the door.

My defiance and defences gave the attendants the excuse for which they had said they were waiting; and my success in keeping them out for two or three minutes only served to enrage them. By the time they had gained entrance they had become furies. One was a young man of twenty-seven. Physically he was a fine specimen of manhood; morally he was deficient—thanks to the dehumanizing effect of several years in the employ of different institutions whose officials countenanced improper methods of care and treatment. It was he who now attacked me in the dark of my prison room. The head attendant stood by, holding a lantern which shed a dim light.

The door once open, I offered no further resistance. First I was knocked down. Then for several minutes I was kicked about the room—struck, kneed and choked. My assailant even attempted to grind his heel into my cheek. In this he failed, for

I was there protected by a heavy beard which I wore at that time. But my shins, elbows, and back were cut by his heavy shoes; and had I not instinctively drawn up my knees to my elbows for the protection of my body, I might have been seriously, perhaps fatally, injured. As it was, I was severely cut and bruised. When my strength was nearly gone, I feigned unconsciousness. This ruse alone saved me from further punishment, for usually a premeditated assault is not ended until the patient is mute and helpless. When they had accomplished their purpose, they left me huddled in a corner to wear out the night as best I might—to live or die for all they cared.

Strange as it may seem, I slept well. But not at once. Within five minutes I was busily engaged writing an account of the assault. A trained war correspondent could not have pulled himself together in less time. As usual I had recourse to my bit of contraband lead pencil, this time a pencil which had been smuggled to me the very first day of my confinement by a sympathetic fellow-patient. When he had pushed under my cell door that little implement of war, it had loomed as large in my mind as a battering-ram. Paper I had none; but I had previously found walls to be a fair substitute. I therefore now selected and wrote upon a rectangular spot—about three feet by two—which marked the reflection of a light in the corridor just outside my transom.

The next morning, when the assistant physician appeared, he was accompanied as usual by the guilty head attendant who, on the previous night, had held the lantern.

"Doctor," I said, "I have something to tell you,"—and I glanced significantly at the attendant. "Last night I had a most unusual experience. I have had many imaginary experiences during the past two years and a half, and it may be that last night's was not real. Perhaps the whole thing was phantasmagoric—like what I used to see during the first months of my illness. Whether it was so or not I shall leave you to judge. It just happens to be my impression that I was brutally assaulted last night. If it was a dream, it is the first thing of the kind that ever left visible evidence on my body."

With that I uncovered to the doctor a score of bruises and lacerations. I knew these would be more impressive than any words of mine. The doctor put on a knowing look, but said nothing and soon left the room. His guilty subordinate tried to appear unconcerned, and I really believed he thought me not absolutely sure of the events of the previous night, or at least unaware of his share in them.

∞XXI∞

Neither of the attendants involved in the assault upon me was discharged. This fact made me more eager to gain wider knowledge of conditions. The self-control which had enabled me to suspend speech for a whole day now stood me in good stead. It enabled me to avert much suffering that would have been my portion had I been like the majority of my ward-mates. Time and again I surrendered when an attendant was about to chastise me. But at least a score of patients in the ward were not so well equipped mentally, and these were viciously assaulted again and again by the very men who had so thoroughly initiated me into the mysteries of their black art.

I soon observed that the only patients who were not likely to be subjected to abuse were the very ones least in need of care and treatment. The violent, noisy, and troublesome patient was abused because he was violent, noisy, and troublesome. The patient too weak, physically or mentally, to attend to his own wants was frequently abused because of that very helplessness which made it necessary for the attendants to wait upon him.

Usually a restless or troublesome patient placed in the violent ward was assaulted the very first day. This procedure seemed to be a part of the established code of dishonor. The attendants imagined that the best way to gain control of a patient was to cow him from the first. In fact, these fellows—nearly all of them ignorant and untrained—seemed to believe that "violent could not be handled in any other way. One attendant, the very day he had been discharged for choking a patient into an insensibility so profound that it had been necessary to call a physician to restore him, said to me, "They are getting pretty damned strict these days, discharging a man simply for choking a patient." This illustrates the attitude of many attendants. On the other hand, that the discharged employé soon secured a position in a similar institution not twenty miles distant illustrates the attitude of some hospital managements.

I recall the advent of a new attendant—a young man studying to become a physician. At first he seemed inclined to treat patients kindly, but he soon fell into brutal ways. His change of heart was due partly to the brutalizing environment, but more directly to the attitude of the three hardened attendants who mistook his consideration for cowardice and taunted him for it. Just to prove his mettle he began to assault patients, and one day knocked me down simply for refusing to stop my prattle at his command. That the environment in some institutions is brutalizing, was strikingly shown in the testimony of an attendant at a public investigation in Kentucky, who said, "When I came here, if anyone had told me I would be guilty of striking patients I would have called him crazy himself, but now I take delight in punching hell out of them."

I found that an unnecessary and continued lack of outdoor exercise tended to multiply deeds of violence. Patients were supposed to be taken for a walk at least once a day, and twice, when the weather permitted. Yet those in the violent ward (and it was they who most need the exercise) usually got out of doors only when the attendants saw fit to take them. For weeks a ward-mate—a man sane enough to enjoy freedom, had he had a home to go to—kept a record of the number of our walks. It showed that we averaged not more than one or two a week for a period of two months. This, too, in the face of many pleasant days, which made the close confinement doubly irksome. The lazy fellows on whose leisure we waited preferred to remain in the ward, playing cards, smoking, and telling their kind of stories. The attendants needed regular exercise quite as much as the patients and when they failed to employ their energy in this healthful way, they were likely to use it at the expense of the bodily comfort of their helpless charges.

If lack of exercise produced a need of discipline, each disciplinary move, on the other hand, served only to inflame us the more. Some wild animals can be clubbed into a semblance of obedience, yet it is a treacherous obedience at best, and justly so. And that is the only kind of obedience into which a *man* can be clubbed. To imagine otherwise of a human being, sane or insane, is the very essence of insanity itself. A temporary leisure may be won for the aggressor, but in the long run he will be put to greater inconvenience than he would be by a more humane method. It was repression and wilful frustration of reasonable desires which kept me a seeming maniac and made seeming maniacs of others. Whenever I was released from lock and key and permitted to mingle with the so-called violent patients, I was surprised to find that comparatively few were by nature troublesome or noisy. A patient, calm in mind and passive in behavior three hundred and sixty days in the year, may, on one of the remaining days, commit some slight transgression, or, more likely, be goaded into one by an attendant or needlessly led into one by a tactless physician. His indiscretion may consist merely in an unmannerly announcement to the doctor of how lightly the latter is regarded by the patient. At once he is banished to the violent ward, there to remain for weeks, perhaps indefinitely.

Like fires and railroad disasters, assaults seemed to come in groups. Days would pass without a single outbreak. Then would come a veritable carnival of abuse—due almost invariably to the attendants' state of mind, not to an unwonted aggressiveness on the part of the patients. I can recall as especially noteworthy several instances of atrocious abuse. Five patients were chronic victims. Three of them, peculiarly irresponsible, suffered with especial regularity, scarcely a day passing without bringing to them its quota of punishment. One of these, almost an idiot, and quite too inarticulate to tell a convincing story even under the most favorable conditions, became so cowed that, whenever an attendant passed, he would circle his oppressor as a whipped cur circles a cruel master. If this avoidance became too marked, the attendant would then and there chastise him for the implied, but unconscious insult.

There was a young man, occupying a cell next to mine in the Bull Pen, who was so far out of his mind as to be absolutely irresponsible. His offence was that he could not comprehend and obey. Day after day I could hear the blows and kicks as they fell upon his body, and his incoherent cries for mercy were as painful to hear as they are impossible to forget. That he survived is surprising. What wonder that this man, who was "violent," or who was made violent, would not permit the attendants to dress him! But he had a half-witted friend, a ward-mate, who could coax him into his clothes when his oppressors found him most intractable.

Of all the patients known to me, the one who was assaulted with the greatest frequency was an incoherent and irresponsible man of sixty years. This patient was restless and forever talking or shouting, as any man might if oppressed by such delusions as his. He was profoundly convinced that one of the patients had stolen his stomach—an idea inspired perhaps by the remarkable corpulency of the person accused. His loss he would woefully voice even while eating. Of course, argument to the contrary had no effect; and his monotonous recital of his imaginary troubles made him unpopular with those whose business it was to care for him. They showed him no mercy. Each day—including the hours of the night, when the night watch took a hand—he was belabored with fists, broom handles, and frequently with the heavy bunch of keys which attendants usually carry on a long chain. He was also kicked and choked, and his suffering was aggravated by his almost continuous confinement in the Bull Pen. An exception to the general rule (for such continued abuse often causes death), this man lived a long time—five years, as I learned later.

Another victim, forty-five years of age, was one who had formerly been a successful man of affairs. His was a forceful personality, and the traits of his sane days influenced his conduct when he broke down mentally. He was in the expansive phase of paresis, a phase distinguished by an exaggerated sense of well-being, and by delusions of grandeur which are symptoms of this form as well as of several other forms of mental disease. Paresis, as everyone knows, is considered incurable and victims of it seldom live more than three or four years. In this instance, instead of trying to make the patient's last days comfortable, the attendants subjected him to a course of treatment severe enough to have sent even a sound man to an early grave. I endured privations and severe abuse for one month at the State Hospital. This man suffered in all ways worse treatment for many months.

I became well acquainted with two jovial and witty Irishmen. They were common laborers. One was a hod carrier, and a strapping fellow. When he arrived at the institution, he was at once placed in the violent ward, though his "violence" consisted of nothing more than an annoying sort of irresponsibility. He irritated the attendants by persistently doing certain trivial things after they had been forbidden. The attendants made no allowance for his condition of mind. His repetition of a forbidden act was interpreted as deliberate disobedience. He was physically powerful, and they determined to cow him. Of the master assault by which they attempted to do this I was not an eyewitness. But I was an ear witness. It was committed behind a closed door; and I heard the dull thuds of the blows, and I heard the cries for mercy until there was no breath left in the man with which he could beg even for his life. For days, that wrecked Hercules dragged himself about the ward moaning pitifully. He complained of pain in his side and had difficulty in breathing, which would seem to indicate that some of his ribs had been fractured. This man was often punished, frequently for complaining of the torture already inflicted. But later, when he began to return to the normal, his good-humor and native wit won for him an increasing degree of good treatment.

The other patient's arch offence—a symptom of his disease—was that he gabbled incessantly. He could no more stop talking than he could right his reason on command. Yet his failure to become silent at a word was the signal for punishment. On one occasion an attendant ordered him to stop talking and take a seat at the further end of the corridor, about forty feet distant. He was doing his best to obey, even running to keep ahead of the attendant at his heels. As they passed the spot where I was sitting, the attendant felled him with a blow behind the ear; and, in falling, the patient's head barely missed the wall.

Addressing me, the attendant said, "Did you see that?"

"Yes," I replied, "and I'll not forget it."

"Be sure to report it to the doctor," he said, which remark showed his contempt, not only for me, but for those in authority.

The man who had so terribly beaten me was particularly flagrant in ignoring the claims of age. On more than one occasion he viciously attacked a man of over fifty, who, however, seemed much older. He was a Yankee sailing-master, who in his prime could have thrashed his tormentor with ease. But now he was helpless and could only submit. However, he was not utterly abandoned by his old world. His wife called often to see him; and, because of his condition, she was permitted to visit him in his room. Once she arrived a few hours after he had been cruelly beaten. Naturally she asked the attendants how he had come by the hurts—the blackened eye and bruised head. True to the code, they lied. The good wife, perhaps herself a Yankee, was not thus to be fooled; and her growing belief that her husband had been assaulted was confirmed by a sight she saw before her visit was ended. Another patient, a foreigner who was a target for abuse, was knocked flat two or three times as he was roughly forced along the corridor. I saw this little affair and I saw that the good wife saw it. The next day she called again and took her husband home. The result was that after a few (probably sleepless) nights, she had to return him to the hospital and trust to God rather than the State to protect him.

Another victim was a man sixty years of age. He was quite inoffensive, and no patient in the ward seemed to attend more strictly to his own business. Shortly after my transfer from the violent ward this man was so viciously attacked that his arm was broken. The attendant (the man who had so viciously assaulted me) was summarily discharged. Unfortunately, however, the relief afforded the insane was slight and brief, for this same brute, like another whom I have mentioned, soon secured a position in another institution—this one, however, a thousand miles distant.

Death by violence in a violent ward is after all not an unnatural death—for a violent ward. The patient of whom I am about to speak was also an old man—over sixty. Both physically and mentally he was a wreck. On being brought to the institution he was at once placed in the Bull Pen, probably because of his previous history of violence while at his own home. But his violence (if it ever existed) had already spent itself, and had come to be nothing more than an utter incapacity to obey. His offence was that he was too weak to attend to his common wants. The day after his arrival, shortly before noon, he lay stark naked and helpless upon the bed in his cell. This I know, for I went to investigate immediately after a ward-mate had informed me of the vicious way in which the head attendant had assaulted the sick man. My informant was a man whose word regarding an incident of this character I would take as readily as that of any man I know. He came to me, knowing that I had taken upon myself the duty of reporting such abominations. My informant feared to take the initiative, for, like many other patients who believe themselves doomed to continued confinement, he feared to invite abuse at the hands of vengeful attendants. I therefore promised him that I would report the case as soon as I had an opportunity.

All day long this victim of an attendant's unmanly passion lay in his cell in what seemed to be a semi-conscious condition. I took particular pains to observe his condition, for I felt that the assault of the morning might result in death. That night, after the doctor's regular tour of inspection, the patient in question was transferred to a room next my own. The mode of transfer impressed itself upon my memory. Two attendants— one of them being he who had so brutally beaten the patient— placed the man in a sheet and, each taking an end, carried the hammocklike contrivance, with its inert contents, to what proved to be its last resting-place above ground. The bearers seemed as much concerned about their burden as one might be about a dead dog, weighted and ready for the river.

That night the patient died. Whether he was murdered none can ever know. But it is my honest opinion that he was. Though he might never have recovered, it is plain that he would have lived days, perhaps months. And had he been humanely, nay, scientifically, treated, who can say that he might not have been restored to health and home?

The young man who had been my companion in mischief in the violent ward was also terribly abused. I am sure I do not exaggerate when I say that on ten occasions, within a period of two months, this man was cruelly assaulted, and I do not know how many times he suffered assaults of less severity. After one of these chastisements, I asked him why he persisted in his petty transgressions when he knew that he thereby invited such body-racking abuse.

"Oh," he said, laconically, "I need the exercise."

To my mind, the man who, with such gracious humor, could refer to what was in reality torture deserved to live a century. But an unkind fate decreed that he should die young. Ten months after his commitment to the State Hospital he was discharged as improved—but not cured. This was not an unusual procedure; nor was it in his case apparently an unwise one, for he seemed fit for freedom. During the first month of regained liberty, he hanged himself. He left no message of excuse. In my opinion, none was necessary. For aught any man knows, the memories of the abuse, torture, and injustice which were so long his portion may have proved to be the last straw which overbalanced the desire to live.

Patients with less stamina than mine often submitted with meekness; and none so aroused my sympathy as those whose submission was due to the consciousness that they had no relatives or friends to support them in a fight for their rights. On behalf of these, with my usual piece of smuggled lead pencil, I soon began to indite and submit to the officers of the institution, letters in which I described the cruel practices which came under my notice. My reports were perfunctorily accepted and at once forgotten or ignored. Yet these letters, so far as they related to overt acts witnessed, were lucid and should have been convincing. Furthermore, my allegations were frequently corroborated by bruises on the bodies of the patients. My usual custom was to write an account of each assault and hand it to the doctor in authority. Frequently I would submit these reports to the attendants with instructions first to read and then deliver them to the superintendent or the assistant physician. The men whose cruelty I thus laid bare read with evident but perverted pleasure my accounts of assaults, and laughed and joked about my ineffectual attempts to bring them to book.

❦XXIII❧

I refused to be a martyr. Rebellion was my watchword. The only difference between the doctor's opinion of me and mine of him was that he could refuse utterance to his thoughts. Yes— there was another difference. Mine could be expressed only in words—his in grim acts.

I repeatedly made demands for those privileges to which I knew I was entitled. When he saw fit to grant them, I gave him perfunctory thanks. When he refused—as he usually did—I at once poured upon his head the vials of my wrath. One day I would be on the friendliest terms with the doctor, the next I would upbraid him for some denial of my rights—or, as frequently happened, for not intervening in behalf of the rights of others.

It was after one of these wrangles that I was placed in a cold cell in the Bull Pen at eleven o'clock one morning. Still without shoes and with no more covering than underclothes, I was forced to stand, sit, or lie upon a bare floor as hard and cold as the pavement outside. Not until sundown was I provided even with a drugget, and this did little good, for already I had become thoroughly chilled. In consequence I contracted a severe cold which added greatly to my discomfort and might have led to serious results had I been of less sturdy fibre.

This day was the thirteenth of December and the twenty-second of my exile in the violent ward. I remember it distinctly for it was the seventy-seventh birthday of my father, to whom I wished to write a congratulatory letter. This had been my custom for years when absent from home on that anniversary. And well do I remember when, and under what conditions, I asked the doctor for permission. It was night. I was flat on my drugget-bed. My cell was lighted only by the feeble rays of a lantern held by an attendant to the doctor on this his regular visit. At first I couched my request in polite language. The doctor merely refused to grant it. I then put forth my plea in a way calculated to arouse sympathy. He remained unmoved. I then pointed out that he was defying the law of the State which provided that a patient should have stationery—a statute, the spirit of which at least meant that he should be permitted to communicate with his conservator. It was now three weeks since I had been permitted to write or send a letter to anyone. Contrary to my custom, therefore, I made my final demand in the form of a concession. I promised that I would write only a conventional note of congratulation, making no mention whatever of my plight. It was a fair offer; but to accept it would have been an implied admission that there was something to conceal, and for this, if for no other reason, it was refused.

Thus, day after day, I was repressed in a manner which probably would have driven many a sane man to violence. Yet the doctor would frequently exhort me to play the gentleman. Were good manners and sweet submission ever the product of such treatment? Deprived of my clothes, of sufficient food, of warmth, of all sane companionship and of my liberty, I told those in authority that so long as they should continue to treat me as the vilest of criminals, I should do my best to complete the illusion. The burden of proving my sanity was placed upon me. I was told that so soon as I became polite and meek and lowly I should find myself in possession of my clothes and of certain privileges. In every instance I must earn my reward before being entrusted with it. If the doctor, instead of demanding of me all the negative virtues in the catalogue of spineless saints, had given me my clothes on the condition that they would be taken from me again if I so much as removed a button, his course would doubtless have been productive of good results. Thus I might have had my clothes three weeks earlier than I did, and so been spared much suffering from the cold.

I clamored daily for a lead pencil. This little luxury represents the margin of happiness for hundreds of the patients, just as a plug or package of tobacco represents the margin of happiness for thousands of others; but for seven weeks no doctor or attendant gave me one. To be sure, by reason of my somewhat exceptional persistence and ingenuity, I managed to be always in possession of some substitute for a pencil, surreptitiously obtained, a fact which no doubt had something to do with the doctor's indifference to my request. But my inability to secure a pencil in a legitimate way was a needless source of annoyance to me, and many of my verbal indiscretions were directly inspired by the doctor's continued refusal.

It was an assistant physician, other than the one regularly in charge of my case, who at last relented and presented me with a good, whole lead pencil. By so doing he placed himself high on my list of benefactors; for that little shaftlike implement, magnified by my lively appreciation, became as the very axis of the earth.

❧XXIV☙

A few days before Christmas my most galling deprivation was at last removed. That is, my clothes were restored. These I treated with great respect. Not so much as a thread did I destroy. Clothes, as is known, have a sobering and civilizing effect, and from the very moment I was again provided with presentable outer garments my conduct rapidly improved. The assistant physician with whom I had been on such variable terms of friendship and enmity even took me for a sleigh-ride. With this improvement came other privileges or, rather, the granting of my rights. Late in December I was permitted to send letters to my conservator. Though some of my blood-curdling letters were confiscated, a few detailing my experiences were forwarded. The account of my sufferings naturally distressed my conservator, but, as he said when he next visited me: "What could I have done to help you? If the men in this State whose business it is to run these institutions cannot manage you, I am at a loss to know what to do." True, he could have done little or nothing, for he did not then know the ins and outs of the baffling situation into which the ties of blood had drawn him.

About the middle of January the doctor in charge of my case went for a two weeks' vacation. During his absence an older member of the staff took charge of the violent ward. A man of wider experience and more liberal ideas than his predecessor, he at once granted me several real privileges. One day he permitted me to pay a brief visit to the best ward—the one from which I had been transferred two months earlier. I thus was able again to mingle with many seemingly normal men, and though I enjoyed this privilege upon but one occasion, and then only for a few hours, it gave me intense satisfaction.

Altogether the last six weeks of the fourteen during which I was confined in the violent ward were comfortable and relatively happy. I was no longer subjected to physical abuse, though this exemption was largely due to my own skill in avoiding trouble. I was no longer cold and hungry. I was allowed a fair amount of outdoor exercise which, after my close confinement, proved to be a delightful shock. But, above all, I was again given an adequate supply of stationery and drawing materials, which became as tinder under the focussed rays of my artistic eagerness. My mechanical investigations were gradually set aside. Art and literature again held sway. Except when out of doors taking my allotted exercise, I remained in my room reading, writing, or drawing. This room of mine soon became a Mecca for the most irrepressible and loquacious characters in the ward. But I soon schooled myself to shut my ears to the incoherent prattle of my unwelcome visitors. Occasionally, some of them would become obstreperous—perhaps because of my lordly order to leave the room. Often did they threaten to throttle me; but I ignored the threats, and they were never carried out. Nor was I afraid that they would be. Invariably I induced them to obey.

The drawings I produced at this time were crude. For the most part they consisted of copies of illustrations which I had cut from magazines that had miraculously found their way into the violent ward. The heads of men and women interested me most, for I had decided to take up portraiture. At first I was content to draw in black and white, but soon I procured some colors and from that time on devoted my attention to mastering pastel.

In the world of letters I had made little progress. My compositions were for the most part epistles addressed to relatives and friends and to those in authority at the hospital. Frequently the letters addressed to the doctors were sent in sets of three—this to save time, for I was very busy. The first letter of such a series would contain my request, couched in friendly and polite terms. To this I would add a postscript, worded about as follows: "If, after reading this letter, you feel inclined to refuse my request, please read letter number two." Letter number two would be severely formal—a businesslike repetition of the request made in letter number one. Again a postscript would advise the reader to consult letter number three, if the reading of number two had failed to move him. Letter number three was invariably a brief philippic in which I would consign the unaccommodating doctor to oblivion.

In this way I expended part of my prodigious supply of feeling and energy. But I had also another way of reducing my creative pressure. Occasionally, from sheer excess of emotion, I would burst into verse, of a quality not to be doubted. Of that quality the reader shall judge, for I am going to quote a "creation" written under circumstances which, to say the least, were adverse. Before writing these lines I had never attempted verse in my life—barring intentionally inane doggerel. And, as I now judge these lines, it is probably true that even yet I have never written a poem. Nevertheless, my involuntary, almost automatic outburst is at least suggestive of the fervor that was in me. These fourteen lines were written within thirty minutes of the time I first conceived the idea; and I present them substantially as they first took form. From a psychological standpoint at least, I am told, they are not without interest.

LIGHT

Man's darkest hour is the hour before he's born,
Another is the hour just before the Dawn;
From Darkness unto Life and Light he leaps,
To Life but once,—to Light as oft as God wills he should.
'Tis God's own secret, why
Some live long, and others early die;
For Life depends on Light, and Light on God,
Who hath given to Man the perfect knowledge
That Grim Despair and Sorrow end in Light
And Life everlasting, in realms
Where darkest Darkness becomes Light;
But not the Light Man knows,
Which only is Light
Because God told Man so.

These verses, which breathe religion, were written in an environment which was anything but religious. With curses of ward-mates ringing in my ears, some subconscious part of me seemed to force me to write at its dictation. I was far from being in a pious frame of mind myself, and the quality of my thought surprised me then—as it does now.

❧XXV☙

Though I continued to respect my clothes, I did not at once cease to tear such material as would serve me in my scientific investigations. Gravity being conquered, it was inevitable that I should devote some of my time to the invention of a flying-machine. This was soon perfected—in my mind; and all I needed, that I might test the device, was my liberty. As usual I was unable to explain how I should produce the result which I so confidently foretold. But I believed and proclaimed that I should, ere long, fly to St. Louis and claim and receive the one-hundred-thousand-dollar reward offered by the Commission of the Louisiana Purchase Exposition for the most efficient airship to be exhibited. The moment the thought winged its way through my mind, I had not only a flying-machine, but a fortune in the bank. Being where I could not dissipate my riches, I became a lavish verbal spender. I was in a mood to buy anything, and I whiled away many an hour planning what to do with my fortune. The St. Louis prize was a paltry trifle. I reasoned that the man who could harness gravity had at his beck and call the world and all that therein is. This sudden accession of wealth made my vast humanitarian projects seem only the more feasible. What could be more delightful, I thought, than the furnishing and financing of ideas of a magnitude to stagger humanity. My condition was one of ecstatic suspense. Give me my liberty and I would show a sleepy old world what could be done to improve conditions, not only among the insane, but along every line of beneficent endeavor.

The city of my birth was to be made a garden-spot. All defiling, smoke-begriming factories were to be banished to an innocuous distance. Churches were to give way to cathedrals; the city itself was to become a paradise of mansions. Yale University was to be transformed into the most magnificent—yet efficient—seat of learning in the world. For once, college professors were to be paid adequate salaries, and alluring provision for their declining years was to be made. New Haven should become a very hotbed of culture. Art galleries, libraries, museums and theatres of a dreamlike splendor were to rise whenever and wherever I should will. Why absurd? Was it not I who would defray the cost? The famous buildings of the Old World were to be reproduced, if, indeed, the originals could not be purchased, brought to this country and reassembled. Not far from New Haven there is a sandy plain, once the bed of the Connecticut River, but now a kind of miniature desert. I often smile as I pass it on the train; for it was here, for the edification of those who might never be able to visit the Valley of the Nile, that I planned to erect a pyramid that should out-Cheops the original. My harnessed gravity, I believed, would not only enable me to overcome existing mechanical difficulties, but it would make the quarrying of immense monoliths as easy as the slicing of bread, and the placing of them in position as easy as the laying of bricks.

After all, delusions of grandeur are the most entertaining of toys. The assortment which my imagination provided was a comprehensive one. I had tossed aside the blocks of childhood days. Instead of laboriously piling small squares of wood one upon another in an endeavor to build the tiny semblance of a house, I now, in this second childhood of mine, projected against thin air phantom edifices planned and completed in the twinkling of an eye. To be sure, such houses of cards almost immediately superseded one another, but the vanishing of one could not disturb a mind that had ever another interesting bauble to take its place. And therein lies part of the secret of the happiness peculiar to that stage of elation which is distinguished by delusions of grandeur—always provided that he who is possessed by them be not subjected to privation and abuse. The sane man who can prove that he is rich in material wealth is not nearly so happy as the mentally disordered man whose delusions trick him into believing himself a modern Crœsus. A wealth of Midaslike delusions is no burden. Such a fortune, though a misfortune in itself, bathes the world in a golden glow. No clouds obscure the vision. Optimism reigns supreme. "Failure" and "impossible" are as words from an unknown tongue. And the unique satisfaction about a fortune of this fugitive type is that its loss occasions no regret. One by one the phantom ships of treasure sail away for parts unknown; until, when the last ship has become but a speck on the mental horizon, the observer makes the happy discovery that his pirate fleet has left behind it a priceless wake of Reason!

☙XXVI☙

Early in March, 1902, having lived in a violent ward for nearly four months, I was transferred to another—a ward quite as orderly as the best in the institution, though less attractively furnished than the one in which I had first been placed. Here also I had a room to myself; in this instance, however, the room had not only a bed, but a chair and a wardrobe. With this elaborate equipment I was soon able to convert my room into a veritable studio. Whereas in the violent ward it had been necessary for me to hide my writing and drawing materials to keep other patients from taking them, in my new abode I was able to conduct my literary and artistic pursuits without the annoyances which had been inevitable during the preceding months.

Soon after my transfer to this ward I was permitted to go out of doors and walk to the business section of the city, two miles distant. But on these walks I was always accompanied. To one who has never surrendered any part of his liberty such surveillance would no doubt seem irksome; yet, to me, after being so closely confined, the ever-present attendant seemed a companion rather than a guard. These excursions into the sane and free world were not only a great pleasure, they were almost a tonic. To rub elbows with normal people tended to restore my mental poise. That the casual passer-by had no way of knowing that I was a patient, out for a walk about the city, helped me

155

gain that self-confidence so essential to the success of one about to re-enter a world from which he had long been cut off.

My first trips to the city were made primarily for the purpose of supplying myself with writing and drawing materials. While enjoying these welcome tastes of liberty, on more than one occasion I surreptitiously mailed certain letters which I did not dare entrust to the doctor. Under ordinary circumstances such an act on the part of one enjoying a special privilege would be dishonorable. But the circumstances that then obtained were not ordinary. I was simply protecting myself against what I believed to be unjust and illegal confiscation of letters.

I have already described how an assistant physician arbitrarily denied my request that I be permitted to send a birthday letter to my father, thereby not merely exceeding his authority and ignoring decency, but, consciously or unconsciously, stifling a sane impulse. That this should occur while I was confined in the Bull Pen was, perhaps, not so surprising. But about four months later, while I was in one of the best wards, a similar, though less open, interference occurred. At this time I was so nearly normal that my discharge was a question of but a very few months. Anticipating my return to my old world, I decided to renew former relationships. Accordingly, my brother, at my suggestion, informed certain friends that I should be pleased to receive letters from them. They soon wrote. In the meantime the doctor had been instructed to deliver to me any and all letters that might arrive. He did so for a time, and that without censoring. As was to be expected, after nearly three almost letterless years, I found rare delight in replying to my reawakened correspondents. Yet some of these letters, written for the deliberate purpose of re-establishing myself in the sane world, were destroyed by the doctor in authority. At the time, not one word did he say to me about the matter. I had handed him for mailing certain letters, unsealed. He did not mail them, nor did he forward them to my conservator as he should have done, and had earlier agreed to do with all letters which he could not see his way clear to approve. It was fully a month before I learned that my friends had not received my replies to their letters. Then I accused the doctor of destroying them, and he, with belated frankness, admitted that he had done so. He offered no better excuse than the mere statement that he did not approve of the sentiments I had expressed. Another flagrant instance was that of a letter addressed to me in reply to one of those which I had posted surreptitiously. The person to whom I wrote, a friend of years' standing, later informed me that he had sent the reply. I never received it. Neither did my conservator. Were it not that I feel absolutely sure that the letter in question was received at the hospital and destroyed, I should not now raise this point. But such a point, if raised at all, must of course be made without that direct proof which can come only from the man guilty of an act which in the sane world is regarded as odious and criminal.

I therefore need not dilate on the reasons which made it necessary for me to smuggle, as it were, to the Governor of the State, a letter of complaint and instruction. This letter was written shortly after my transfer from the violent ward. The abuses of that ward were still fresh in my mind, and the memory of distressing scenes was kept vivid by reports reaching me from friends who were still confined there. These private sleuths of mine I talked with at the evening entertainments or at other gatherings. From them I learned that brutality had become more rife, if anything, since I had left the ward. Realizing that my crusade against the physical abuse of patients thus far had proved of no avail, I determined to go over the heads of the doctors and appeal to the ex-officio head of the institution, the Governor of the State.

On March 12th, 1903, I wrote a letter which so disturbed the Governor that he immediately set about an informal investigation of some of my charges. Despite its prolixity, its unconventional form and what, under other circumstances, would be characterized as almost diabolic impudence and familiarity, my letter, as he said months later when I talked with him, "rang true." The writing of it was an easy matter; in fact, so easy, because of the pressure of truth under which I was laboring at the time, that it embodied a compelling spontaneity.

The mailing of it was not so easy. I knew that the only sure way of getting my thoughts before the Governor was to do my own mailing. Naturally no doctor could be trusted to send an indictment against himself and his colleagues to the one man in the State who had the power to institute such an investigation as might make it necessary for all to seek employment elsewhere. In my frame of mind, to wish to mail my letter was to know how to accomplish the wish. The letter was in reality a booklet. I had thoughtfully used waterproof India drawing ink in writing it, in order, perhaps, that a remote posterity might not be deprived of the document. The booklet consisted of thirty-two eight-by-ten-inch pages of heavy white drawing paper. These I sewed together. In planning the form of my letter I had forgotten to consider the slot of a letter-box of average size. Therefore I had to adopt an unusual method of getting the letter into the mails. My expedient was simple. There was in the town a certain shop where I traded. At my request the doctor gave me permission to go there for supplies. I was of course accompanied by an attendant who little suspected what was under my vest. To conceal and carry my letter in that place had been easy; but to get rid of it after reaching my goal was another matter. Watching my opportunity, I slipped the missive between the leaves of a copy of the *Saturday Evening Post*. This I did, believing that some purchaser would soon discover the letter and mail it. Then I left the shop.

On the back of the wrapper I had endorsed the following words:

"Mr. Postmaster: This package is unsealed. Nevertheless it is first-class matter. Everything I write is necessarily first class. I have affixed two two-cent stamps. If extra postage is needed you will do the Governor a favor if you will put the extra postage on. Or affix 'due' stamps, and let the Governor pay his own bills, as he can well afford to. If you want to know who I am, just ask his Excellency, and oblige,

Yours truly,
?"

Flanking this notice, I had arrayed other forceful sentiments, as follows—taken from statutes which I had framed for the occasion:

"Any person finding a letter or package—duly stamped and addressed—*must* mail same as said letter or package is really in hands of the Government the moment the stamp is affixed."

And again:

"Failure to comply with Federal Statute which forbids any one except addressee to open a letter renders one liable to imprisonment in State Prison."

My letter reached the Governor. One of the clerks at the shop in which I left the missive found and mailed it. From him I afterwards learned that my unique instructions had piqued his curiosity, as well as compelled my wished-for action. Assuming that the reader's curiosity may likewise have been piqued, I shall quote certain passages from this four-thousand-word epistle of protest. The opening sentence read as follows: "If you have had the courage to read the above" (referring to an unconventional heading) "I hope you will read on to the end of this epistle—thereby displaying real Christian fortitude and learning a few facts which I think should be brought to your attention."

I then introduced myself, mentioning a few common friends, by way of indicating that I was not without influential political connections, and proceeded as follows: "I take pleasure in informing you that I am in the Crazy Business and am holding my job down with ease and a fair degree of grace. Being in the Crazy Business, I understand certain phases of the business about which you know nothing. You as Governor are at present 'head devil' in this 'hell,' though I know you are unconsciously acting as 'His Majesty's' 1st Lieutenant."

I then launched into my arraignment of the treatment of the insane. The method, I declared, was "wrong from start to finish. The abuses existing here exist in every other institution of the kind in the country. They are all alike—though some of them are of course worse than others. Hell is hell the world over, and I might also add that hell is only a great big bunch of disagreeable details anyway. That's all an Insane Asylum is. If you don't believe it, just go crazy and take up your abode here. In writing this letter I am laboring under no mental excitement. I am no longer subjected to the abuses about which I complain. I am well and happy. In fact I never was so happy as I am now. Whether I am in perfect mental health or not, I shall leave for you to decide. If I am insane today I hope I may never recover my Reason."

First I assailed the management of the private institution where I had been strait-jacketed and referred to "Jekyll-Hyde" as "Dr. —— ——, M.D. (Mentally Deranged)." Then followed an account of the strait-jacket experience; then an account of abuses at the State Hospital. I described in detail the most brutal assault that fell to my lot. In summing up I said, "The attendants claimed next day that I had called them certain names. Maybe I did—though I don't believe I did at all. What of it? This is no young ladies' boarding school. Should a man be nearly killed because he swears at attendants who swear like pirates? I have seen at least fifteen men, many of them mental and physical wrecks, assaulted just as brutally as I was, and usually without a cause. I know that men's lives have been shortened by these brutal assaults. And that is only a polite way of saying that murder has been committed here." Turning next to the matter of the women's wards, I said: "A patient in this ward—a man in his right mind, who leaves here on Tuesday next—told me that a woman patient told him that she had seen many a helpless woman dragged along the floor by her hair, and had also seen them choked by attendants who used a wet towel as a sort of garrote. I have been through the mill and believe every word of the abuse. You will perhaps doubt it, as it seems impossible. Bear in mind, though, that everything bad and disagreeable is possible in an Insane Asylum."

It will be observed that I was shrewd enough to qualify a charge I could not prove.

When I came to the matter of the Bull Pen, I wasted no words: "The Bull Pen," I wrote, "is a pocket edition of the New York Stock Exchange during a panic."

I next pointed out the difficulties a patient must overcome in mailing letters: "It is impossible for any one to send a letter to you *via* the office. The letter would be consigned to the wastebasket—unless it was a particularly crazy letter—in which case it might reach you, as you would then pay no attention to it. But a sane letter and a *true* letter, telling about the abuses which exist here would stand no show of being mailed. The way in which mail is tampered with by the medical staff is contemptible."

I then described my stratagem in mailing my letter to the Governor. Discovering that I had left a page of my epistolary booklet blank, I drew upon it a copy of Rembrandt's Anatomy Lesson, and under it wrote: "This page was skipped by mistake. Had to fight fifty-three days to get writing paper and I hate to waste any space—hence the masterpiece—drawn in five minutes. Never drew a line till September 26 (last) and never took lessons in my life. I think you will readily believe my statement." Continuing in the same half-bantering vein, I said: "I intend to immortalize all members of medical staff of State Hospital for Insane—when I illustrate my Inferno, which, when written, will make Dante's Divine Comedy look like a French Farce."

I then outlined my plans for reform: "Whether my suggestions meet with approval or not," I wrote, "will not affect the result—though opposition on your part would perhaps delay reforms. I have decided to devote the next few years of my life to correcting abuses now in existence in every asylum in this country. I know how these abuses can be corrected and I intend —later on, when I understand the subject better—to draw up a Bill of Rights for the Insane. Every State in the Union will pass it, because it will be founded on the Golden Rule. I am desirous of having the co-operation of the Governor of Connecticut, but if my plans do not appeal to him I shall deal directly with his only superior, the President of the United States. When Theodore Roosevelt hears my story his blood will boil. I would write to him now, but I am afraid he would jump in and correct abuses too quickly. And by doing it too quickly too little good would be accomplished."

Waxing crafty, yet, as I believed, writing truth, I continued: "I need money badly, and if I cared to, I could sell my information and services to the *New York World* or *New York Journal* for a large amount. But I do not intend to advertise Connecticut as a Hell-hole of Iniquity, Insanity, and Injustice. If the facts appeared in the public press at this time, Connecticut would lose caste with her sister States. And they would profit by Connecticut's disgrace and correct the abuses before they could be put on the rack. As these conditions prevail throughout the country, there is no reason why Connecticut should get all the abuse and criticism which would follow any such revelation of disgusting abuse; such inhuman treatment of human wrecks. If publicity is necessary to force you to act—and I am sure it will not be necessary—I shall apply for a writ of habeas corpus, and, in proving my sanity to a jury, I shall incidentally prove your own incompetence. Permitting such a whirlwind reformer to drag Connecticut's disgrace into open court would prove your incompetence."

For several obvious reasons it is well that I did not at that time attempt to convince a jury that I was mentally sound. The mere outlining of my ambitious scheme for reform would have caused my immediate return to the hospital. That scheme, however, was a sound and feasible one, as later events have proved. But, taking hold of me, as it did, while my imagination was at white heat, I was impelled to attack my problem with compromising energy and, for a time, in a manner so unconvincing as to obscure the essential sanity of my cherished purpose.

I closed my letter as follows: "No doubt you will consider certain parts of this letter rather 'fresh.' I apologize for any such passages now, but, as I have an Insane License, I do not hesitate to say what I think. What's the use when one is caged like a criminal?

"P.S. This letter is a confidential one—and is to be returned to the writer upon demand."

The letter was eventually forwarded to my conservator and is now in my possession.

As a result of my protest the Governor immediately interrogated the superintendent of the institution where "Jekyll-Hyde" had tortured me. Until he laid before the superintendent my charges against his assistant, the doctor in authority had not even suspected that I had been tortured. This superintendent took pride in his institution. He was sensitive to criticism and it was natural that he should strive to palliate the offence of his subordinate. He said that I was a most troublesome patient, which was, indeed, the truth; for I had always a way of my own for doing the things that worried those in charge of me. In a word, I brought to bear upon the situation what I have previously referred to as "an uncanny admixture of sanity."

The Governor did not meet the assistant physician who had maltreated me. The reprimand, if there was to be any, was left to the superintendent to administer.

In my letter to the Governor I had laid more stress upon the abuses to which I had been subjected at this private institution than I had upon conditions at the State Hospital where I was when I wrote to him. This may have had some effect on the action he took, or rather failed to take. At any rate, as to the State Hospital, no action was taken. Not even a word of warning was sent to the officials, as I later learned; for before leaving the institution I asked them.

Though my letter did not bring about an investigation, it was not altogether without results. Naturally, it was with considerable satisfaction that I informed the doctors that I had outwitted them, and it was with even greater satisfaction that I now saw those in authority make a determined, if temporary, effort to protect helpless patients against the cruelties of attendants. The moment the doctors were convinced that I had gone over their heads and had sent a characteristic letter of protest to the Governor of the State, that moment they began to protect themselves with an energy born of a realization of their former shortcomings. Whether or not the management in question ever admitted that their unwonted activity was due to my successful stratagem, the fact remains that the summary discharge of several attendants accused and proved guilty of brutality immediately followed and for a while put a stop to wanton assaults against which for a period of four months I had protested in vain. Patients who still lived in the violent ward told me that comparative peace reigned about this time.

ᴥXXVIIᴥ

My failure to force the Governor to investigate conditions at the State Hospital convinced me that I could not hope to prosecute my reforms until I should regain my liberty and re-establish myself in my old world. I therefore quitted the rôle of reformer-militant; and, but for an occasional outburst of righteous indignation at some flagrant abuse which obtruded itself upon my notice, my demeanor was that of one quite content with his lot in life.

I was indeed content—I was happy. Knowing that I should soon regain my freedom, I found it easy to forgive—taking great pains not to forget—any injustice which had been done me. Liberty is sweet, even to one whose appreciation of it has never been augmented by its temporary loss. The pleasurable emotions which my impending liberation aroused within me served to soften my speech and render me more tractable. This change the assistant physician was not slow to note, though he was rather slow in placing in me the degree of confidence which I felt I deserved. So justifiable, however, was his suspicion that even at the time I forgave him for it. I had on so many prior occasions "played possum" that the doctor naturally attributed complex and unfathomable motives to my most innocent acts. For a long time he seemed to think that I was trying to capture his confidence, win the privilege of an unlimited parole, and so effect my escape. Doubtless he had not forgotten the several plans for escape which I had dallied with and bragged about while in the violent ward.

Though I was granted considerable liberty during the months of April, May, and June, 1903, not until July did I enjoy a so-called unlimited parole which enabled me to walk about the neighboring city unattended. My privileges were granted so gradually that these first tastes of regained freedom, though delightful, were not so thrilling as one might imagine. I took everything as a matter of course, and, except when I deliberately analyzed my feelings, was scarcely conscious of my former deprivations.

This power to forget the past—or recall it only at will—has contributed much to my happiness. Some of those who have suffered experiences such as mine are prone to brood upon them, and I cannot but attribute my happy immunity from unpleasant memories to the fact that I have viewed my own case much as a physician might view that of a patient. My past is a thing apart. I can examine this or that phase of it in the clarifying and comforting light of reason, under a memory rendered somewhat microscopic. And I am further compensated by the belief that I have a distinct mission in life—a chance for usefulness that might never have been mine had I enjoyed unbroken health and uninterrupted liberty.

The last few months of my life in the hospital were much alike, save that each succeeding one brought with it an increased amount of liberty. My hours now passed pleasantly. Time did not drag, for I was engaged upon some enterprise every minute. I would draw, read, write, or talk. If any feeling was dominant, it was my feeling for art; and I read with avidity books on the technique of that subject. Strange as it may seem, however, the moment I again found myself in the world of business my desire to become an artist died almost as suddenly as it had been born. Though my artistic ambition was clearly an outgrowth of my abnormal condition, and languished when normality asserted itself, I am inclined to believe I should even now take a lively interest in the study of art if I were so situated as to be deprived of a free choice of my activities. The use of words later enthralled me because so eminently suited to my purposes.

During the summer of 1903, friends and relatives often called to see me. The talks we had were of great and lasting benefit to me. Though I had rid myself of my more extravagant and impossible delusions of grandeur—flying-machines and the like—I still discussed with intense earnestness other schemes, which, though allied to delusions of grandeur, were, in truth, still more closely allied to sanity itself. My talk was of that high, but perhaps suspicious type in which Imagination overrules Common Sense. Lingering delusions, as it were, made great projects seem easy. That they were at least feasible under certain conditions, my mentors admitted. Only I was in an abnormal hurry to produce results. Work that I later realized could not be accomplished in less than five or ten years, if, indeed, in a lifetime, I then believed could be accomplished in a year or two, and by me single-handed. Had I had none but mentally unbalanced people to talk with, I might have continued to cherish a distorted perspective. It was the unanimity of sane opinions that helped me to correct my own views; and I am confident that each talk with relatives and friends hastened my return to normality.

Though I was not discharged from the State Hospital until September 10th, 1903, during the preceding month I visited my home several times, once for three days. These trips were not only interesting, but steadying in effect. I willingly returned to the hospital when my parole expired. Though several friends expressed surprise at this willingness to enter again an institution where I had experienced so many hardships, to me my temporary return was not in the least irksome. As I had penetrated and conquered the mysteries of that dark side of my life, it no longer held any terrors for me. Nor does it to this day. I can contemplate the future with a greater degree of complacency than can some of those whose lot in life has been uniformly fortunate. In fact, I said at that time that, should my condition ever demand it, I would again enter a hospital for the insane, quite as willingly as the average person now enters a hospital for the treatment of bodily ailments.

It was in this complacent and confident mood, and without any sharp line of transition, that I again began life in my old world of companionship and of business.

ᨳXXVIIIᨳ

For the first month of regained freedom I remained at home. These weeks were interesting. Scarcely a day passed that I did not meet several former friends and acquaintances who greeted me as one risen from the dead. And well they might, for my three-year trip among the worlds—rather than around the world—was suggestive of complete separation from the everyday life of the multitude. One profound impression which I received at this time was of the uniform delicacy of feeling exhibited by my well-wishers. In no instance that I can recall was a direct reference made to the nature of my recent illness, until I had first made some remark indicating that I was not averse to discussing it. There was an evident effort on the part of friends and acquaintances to avoid a subject which they naturally supposed I wished to forget. Knowing that their studied avoidance of a delicate subject was inspired by a thoughtful consideration, rather than a lack of interest, I invariably forced the conversation along a line calculated to satisfy a suppressed, but perfectly proper, curiosity which I seldom failed to detect. My decision to stand on my past and look the future in the face, has, I believe, contributed much to my own happiness, and, more than anything else, enabled my friends to view my past as I myself do. By frankly referring to my illness, I put my friends and acquaintances at ease, and at a stroke rid them of that constraint which one must feel in the

169

presence of a person constantly in danger of being hurt by a chance allusion to an unhappy occurrence.

I have said much about the obligation of the sane in reference to easing the burdens of those committed to institutions. I might say almost as much about the attitude of the public toward those who survive such a period of exile, restored, but branded with a suspicion which only time can efface. Though a former patient receives personal consideration, he finds it difficult to obtain employment. No fair-minded man can find fault with this condition of affairs, for an inherent dread of insanity leads to distrust of one who has had a mental breakdown. Nevertheless, the attitude is mistaken. Perhaps one reason for this lack of confidence is to be found in the lack of confidence which a former patient often feels in himself. Confidence begets confidence, and those men and women who survive mental illness should attack their problem as though their absence had been occasioned by any one of the many circumstances which may interrupt the career of a person whose mind has never been other than sound. I can testify to the efficacy of this course, for it is the one I pursued. And I think that I have thus far met with as great a degree of success as I might have reasonably expected had my career never been all but fatally interrupted.

Discharged from the State Hospital in September, 1903, late in October of that same year I went to New York. Primarily my purpose was to study art. I even went so far as to gather information regarding the several schools; and had not my artistic ambition taken wing, I might have worked for recognition in a field where so many strive in vain. But my business instinct, revivified by the commercially surcharged atmosphere of New York, soon gained sway, and within three months I had secured a position with the same firm for which I had worked when I first went to New York six years earlier. It was by the merest chance that I made this most fortunate business connection. By no stretch of my rather elastic imagination can I even now picture a situation that would, at one and the same time, have so perfectly afforded a means of livelihood, leisure in which to indulge my longing to write the story of my experiences, and an opportunity to further my humanitarian project.

Though persons discharged from mental hospitals are usually able to secure, without much difficulty, work as unskilled laborers, or positions where the responsibility is slight, it is often next to impossible for them to secure positions of trust. During the negotiations which led to my employment, I was in no suppliant mood. If anything, I was quite the reverse; and as I have since learned, I imposed terms with an assurance so sublime that any less degree of audacity might have put an end to the negotiations then and there. But the man with whom I was dealing was not only broad-minded, he was sagacious. He recognized immediately such an ability to take care of my own interests as argued an ability to protect those of his firm. But this alone would not have induced the average business man to employ me under the circumstances. It was the common-sense and rational attitude of my employer toward mental illness which determined the issue. This view, which is, indeed, exceptional today, will one day (within a few generations, I believe) be too commonplace to deserve special mention. As the man tersely expressed it: "When an employé is ill, he's ill, and it makes no difference to me whether he goes to a general hospital or a hospital for the insane. Should you ever find yourself in need of treatment or rest, I want you to feel that you can take it when and where you please, and work for us again when you are able."

Dealing almost exclusively with bankers, for that was the nature of my work, I enjoyed almost as much leisure for reading and trying to learn how to write as I should have enjoyed had I had an assured income that would have enabled me to devote my entire time to these pursuits. And so congenial did my work prove, and so many places of interest did I visit, that I might rather have been classed as a "commercial tourist" than as a commercial traveler. To view almost all of the natural wonders and places of historic interest east of the Mississippi, and many west of it; to meet and know representative men and women; to enjoy an almost uninterrupted leisure, and at the same time earn a livelihood—these advantages bear me out in the feeling that in securing the position I did, at the time I did, I enjoyed one of those rare compensations which Fate sometimes bestows upon those who survive unusual adversity.

⊰XXIX⊱

After again becoming a free man, my mind would not abandon the miserable ones whom I had left behind. I thought with horror that my reason had been threatened and baffled at every turn. Without malice toward those who had had me in charge, I yet looked with abhorrence upon the system by which I had been treated. But I realized that I could not successfully advocate reforms in hospital management until I had first proved to relatives and friends my ability to earn a living. And I knew that, after securing a position in the business world, I must first satisfy my employers before I could hope to persuade others to join me in prosecuting the reforms I had at heart. Consequently, during the first year of my renewed business activity (the year 1904), I held my humanitarian project in abeyance and gave all my executive energy to my business duties. During the first half of that year I gave but little time to reading and writing, and none at all to drawing. In a tentative way, however, I did occasionally discuss my project with intimate friends; but I spoke of its consummation as a thing of the uncertain future. At that time, though confident of accomplishing my set purpose, I believed I should be fortunate if my projected book were published before my fortieth year. That I was able to publish it eight years earlier was due to one of those unlooked-for combinations of circumstances which sometimes cause a hurried change of plans.

Late in the autumn of 1904, a slight illness detained me for two weeks in a city several hundred miles from home. The illness itself amounted to little, and, so far as I know, had no direct bearing on later results, except that, in giving me an enforced vacation, it afforded me an opportunity to read several of the world's great books. One of these was "Les Misérables." It made a deep impression on me, and I am inclined to believe it started a train of thought which gradually grew into a purpose so all-absorbing that I might have been overwhelmed by it, had not my over-active imagination been brought to bay by another's common sense. Hugo's plea for suffering Humanity —for the world's miserable—struck a responsive chord within me. Not only did it revive my latent desire to help the afflicted; it did more. It aroused a consuming desire to emulate Hugo himself, by writing a book which should arouse sympathy for and interest in that class of unfortunates in whose behalf I felt it my peculiar right and duty to speak. I question whether anyone ever read "Les Misérables" with keener feeling. By day I read the story until my head ached; by night I dreamed of it.

To resolve to write a book is one thing; to write it—fortunately for the public—is quite another. Though I wrote letters with ease, I soon discovered that I knew nothing of the vigils or methods of writing a book. Even then I did not attempt to predict just when I should begin to commit my story to paper. But, a month later, a member of the firm in whose employ I was made a remark which acted as a sudden spur. One day, while discussing the business situation with me, he informed me that my work had convinced him that he had made no mistake in re-employing me when he did. Naturally I was pleased. I had vindicated his judgment sooner than I had hoped. Aside from appreciating and remembering his compliment, at the time I paid no more attention to it. Not until a fortnight later did the force of his remark exert any peculiar influence on my plans. During that time it apparently penetrated to some subconscious part of me—a part which, on prior occasions, had assumed such authority as to dominate my whole being. But, in this instance, the part that became dominant did not exert an unruly or even unwelcome influence. Full of interest in my business affairs one week, the next I not only had no interest in them, but I had begun even to dislike them. From a matter-of-fact man of business I was transformed into a man whose all-absorbing thought was the amelioration of suffering among the afflicted insane. Travelling on this high plane of ideal humanitarianism, I could get none but a distorted and dissatisfying view of the life I must lead if I should continue to devote my time to the comparatively deadening routine of commercial affairs.

Thus it was inevitable that I should focus my attention on my humanitarian project. During the last week of December I sought ammunition by making a visit to two of the institutions where I had once been a patient. I went there to discuss certain phases of the subject of reform with the doctors in authority. I was politely received and listened to with a degree of deference which was, indeed, gratifying. Though I realized that I was rather intense on the subject of reform, I did not have that clear insight into my state of mind which the doctors had. Indeed, I believe that only those expert in the detection of symptoms of a slightly disturbed mental condition could possibly have observed anything abnormal about me at that time. Only when I discussed my fond project did I betray an abnormal stress of feeling. I could talk as convincingly about business as I had at any time in my life; for even at the height of this wave of enthusiasm I dealt at length with a certain banker who finally placed with my employers a large contract.

After conferring with the doctors, or rather—as it proved—exhibiting myself to them, I returned to New Haven and discussed my project with the President of Yale University. He listened patiently—he could scarcely do otherwise—and did me the great favor of interposing his judgment at a time when I might have made a false move. I told him that I intended to visit Washington at once, to enlist the aid of President Roosevelt; also that of Mr. Hay, Secretary of State. Mr. Hadley tactfully advised me not to approach them until I had more thoroughly crystallized my ideas. His wise suggestion I had the wisdom to adopt.

The next day I went to New York, and on January 1st, 1905, I began to write. Within two days I had written about fifteen thousand words—for the most part on the subject of reforms and how to effect them. One of the documents prepared at that time contained grandiloquent passages that were a portent of coming events—though I was ignorant of the fact. In writing about my project I said, "Whether I am a tool of God or a toy of the devil, time alone will tell; but there will be no misunderstanding Time's answer if I succeed in doing one-tenth of the good things I hope to accomplish. . . . Anything which is feasible in this philanthropic age can easily be put into practice. . . . A listener gets the impression that I hope to do a hundred years' work in a day. They are wrong there, for I'm not so in love with work—as such. I would like though to interest so many people in the accomplishment of my purpose that one hundred years' work might be done in a fraction of that time. Hearty co-operation brings quick results, and once you start a wave of enthusiasm in a sea of humanity, and have for the base of that wave a humanitarian project of great breadth, it will travel with irresistible and ever-increasing impulse to the ends of the earth—which is far enough. According to Dr. ——, many of my ideas regarding the solution of the problem under consideration are years and years in advance of the times. I agree with him, but there is no reason why we should not put 'the times' on board the express train of progress and give civilization a boost to a higher level, until it finally lands on a plateau where performance and perfection will be synonymous terms."

Referring to the betterment of conditions, I said, "And this improvement can never be brought about without some central organization by means of which the best ideas in the world may be crystallized and passed along to those in charge of this army of afflicted ones. The methods to be used to bring about these results must be placed on the same high level as the idea itself. No yellow journalism or other sensational means should be resorted to. Let the thing be worked up secretly and confidentially by a small number of men who know their business. Then when the very best plan has been formulated for the accomplishment of the desired results, and men of money have been found to support the movement until it can take care of itself, announce to the world in a dignified and effective manner the organization and aims of the society, the name of which shall be —, decided later. . . . To start the movement will not require a whole lot of money. It will be started modestly and as financial resources of the society increase, the field will be broadened." . . . "The abuses and correction of same is a mere detail in the general scheme." . . . "It is too early to try to interest anyone in this scheme of preventing breakdowns, as there are other things of more importance to be brought about first—but it will surely come in time."

" 'Uncle Tom's Cabin,' " I continued, "had a very decided effect on the question of slavery of the negro race. Why cannot a book be written which will free the helpless slaves of all creeds and colors confined to-day in the asylums and sanitariums throughout the world? That is, free them from unnecessary abuses to which they are now subjected. Such a book, I believe, can be written and I trust that I may be permitted to live till I am wise enough to write it. Such a book might change the attitude of the public towards those who are unfortunate enough to have the stigma of mental incompetency put upon them. Of course, an insane man is an insane man and while insane should be placed in an institution for treatment, but when that man comes out he should be as free from all taint as the man is who recovers from a contagious disease and again takes his place in society." In conclusion, I said, "From a scientific point of view there is a great field for research. . . . Cannot some of the causes be discovered and perhaps done away with, thereby saving the lives of many—and millions in money? It may come about that some day something will be found which will prevent a complete and incurable mental breakdown. . . ."

Thus did I, as revealed by these rather crude, unrevised quotations, somewhat prophetically, if extravagantly, box the compass that later guided the ship of my hopes (not one of my phantom ships) into a safe channel, and later into a safe harbor.

By way of mental diversion during these creative days at the Yale Club, I wrote personal letters to intimate friends. One of these produced a result unlooked for. There were about it compromising earmarks which the friend to whom it was sent recognized. In it I said that I intended to approach a certain man of wealth and influence who lived in New York, with a view to securing some action that would lead to reform. That was enough. My friend showed the letter to my brother—the one who had acted as my conservator. He knew at once that I was in an excited mental condition. But he could not very well judge the degree of excitement; for when I had last talked with him a week earlier, I had not discussed my larger plans. Business affairs and my hope for business advancement had then alone interested me.

I talked with President Hadley on Friday; Saturday I went to New York; Sunday and Monday I spent at the Yale Club, writing; Tuesday, this telltale letter fell under the prescient eye of my brother. On that day he at once got in touch with me by telephone. We briefly discussed the situation. He did not intimate that he believed me to be in elation. He simply urged me not to attempt to interest anyone in my project until I had first returned to New Haven and talked with him. Now I had already gone so far as to invite my employers to dine with me that very night at the Yale Club for the purpose of informing them of my plans. This I did, believing it to be only fair that they should know what I intended to do, so that they might dispense with my services should they feel that my plans would in any way impair my usefulness as an employé. Of this dinner engagement, therefore, I told my brother. But so insistently did he urge me to defer any such conference as I proposed until I had talked with him that, although it was too late to break the dinner engagement, I agreed to avoid, if possible, any reference to my project. I also agreed to return home the next day.

That night my guests honored me as agreed. For an hour or two we discussed business conditions and affairs in general. Then, one of them referred pointedly to my implied promise to unburden myself on a certain subject, the nature of which he did not at the time know. I immediately decided that it would be best to "take the bull by the horns," submit my plans, and, if necessary, sever my connection with the firm, should its members force me to choose (as I put it) between themselves and Humanity. I then proceeded to unfold my scheme; and, though I may have exhibited a decided intensity of feeling during my discourse, at no time, I believe, did I overstep the bounds of what appeared to be sane enthusiasm. My employers agreed that my purpose was commendable—that no doubt I could and would eventually be able to do much for those I had left behind in a durance I so well knew to be vile. Their one warning was that I seemed in too great a hurry. They expressed the opinion that I had not been long enough re-established in business to be able to persuade people of wealth and influence to take hold of my project. And one of my guests very aptly observed that I could not afford to be a philanthropist, which objection I met by saying that all I intended to do was to supply ideas for those who could afford to apply them. The conference ended satisfactorily. My employers disclaimed any personal objection to my proceeding with my project, if I would, and yet remaining in their employ. They simply urged me to "go slow." "Wait until you're forty," one of them said. I then thought that I might do so. And perhaps I should have waited so long, had not the events of the next two days put me on the right road to an earlier execution of my cherished plans.

The next day, January 4th, true to my word, I went home. That night I had a long talk with my brother. I did not suspect that a man like myself, capable of dealing with bankers and talking for several consecutive hours with his employers without arousing their suspicion as to his mental condition, was to be suspected by his own relatives. Nor, indeed, with the exception of my brother, who had read my suspiciously excellent letter, were any of my relatives disturbed; and he did nothing to disabuse my assurance. After our night conference he left for his own home, casually mentioning that he would see me again the next morning. That pleased me, for I was in a talkative mood and craved an interested listener.

When my brother returned the next morning, I willingly accepted his invitation to go with him to his office, where we could talk without fear of interruption. Arrived there, I calmly sat down and prepared to prove my whole case. I had scarcely "opened fire" when in walked a stranger—a strapping fellow, to whom my brother immediately introduced me. I instinctively felt that it was by no mere chance that this third party had so suddenly appeared. My eyes at once took in the dark blue trousers worn by the otherwise conventionally dressed stranger. That was enough. The situation became so clear that the explanations which followed were superfluous. In a word, I was under arrest, or in imminent danger of being arrested. To say that I was not in the least disconcerted would scarcely be true, for I had not divined my brother's clever purpose in luring me to his office. But I can say, with truth, that I was the coolest person in the room. I knew what I should do next, but my brother and the officer of the law could only guess. The fact is

I did nothing. I calmly remained seated, awaiting the verdict which I well knew my brother, with characteristic decision, had already prepared. With considerable effort—for the situation, he has since told me, was the most trying one of his life—he informed me that on the preceding day he had talked with the doctors to whom I had so opportunely exhibited myself a week earlier. All agreed that I was in a state of elation which might or might not become more pronounced. They had advised that I be persuaded to submit voluntarily to treatment in a hospital, or that I be, if necessary, forcibly committed. On this advice my brother had proceeded to act. And it was well so; for, though I appreciated the fact that I was by no means in a normal state of mind, I had not a clear enough insight into my condition to realize that treatment and a restricted degree of liberty were what I needed, since continued freedom might further inflame an imagination already overwrought.

A few simple statements by my brother convinced me that it was for my own good and the peace of mind of my relatives that I should temporarily surrender my freedom. This I agreed to do. Perhaps the presence of two hundred pounds of brawn and muscle, representing the law, lent persuasiveness to my brother's words. In fact, I did assent the more readily because I admired the thorough, sane, fair, almost artistic manner in which my brother had brought me to bay. I am inclined to believe that, had I suspected that a recommitment was imminent, I should have fled to a neighboring State during the preceding night. Fortunately, however, the right thing was done in the right way at the right time. Though I had been the victim of a clever stratagem, not for one moment thereafter, in any particular, was I deceived. I was frankly told that several doctors had pronounced me elated, and that for my own good I *must* submit to treatment. I was allowed to choose between a probate court commitment which would have "admitted me" to the State Hospital or a "voluntary commitment" which would

enable me to enter the large private hospital where I had previously passed from depression to elation, and had later suffered
tortures. I naturally chose the more desirable of the two dis-
guised blessings, and agreed to start at once for the private
hospital, the one in which I had been when depression gave
way to elation. It was not that I feared again to enter the State
Hospital. I simply wished to avoid the publicity which necessarily would have followed, for at that time the statutes of
Connecticut did not provide for voluntary commitment to the
state hospitals. Then, too, there were certain privileges which I
knew I could not enjoy in a public institution. Having re-
established myself in society and business I did not wish to
forfeit that gain; and as the doctors believed that my period of
elation would be short, it would have been sheer folly to advertise the fact that my mental health had again fallen under
suspicion.

But before starting for the hospital I imposed certain conditions. One was that the man with the authoritative trousers
should walk behind at such a distance that no friend or acquaintance who might see my brother and myself would suspect
that I was under guard; the other was that the doctors at the
institution should agree to grant my every request, no matter
how trivial, so long as doing so could in no way work to my own
injury. My privileges were to include that of reading and writing to my heart's content, and the procuring of such books and
supplies as my fancy might dictate. All this was agreed to. In
return I agreed to submit to the surveillance of an attendant
when I went outside the hospital grounds. This I knew would
contribute to the peace of mind of my relatives, who naturally
could not rid themselves of the fear that one so nearly normal
as myself might take it into his head to leave the State and resist
further attempts at control. As I felt that I could easily elude
my keeper, should I care to escape, his presence also con-

tributed to *my* peace of mind, for I argued that the ability to outwit my guard would atone for the offence itself.

I then started for the hospital; and I went with a willingness surprising even to myself. A cheerful philosophy enabled me to turn an apparently disagreeable situation into one that was positively pleasing to me. I convinced myself that I could extract more real enjoyment from life during the ensuing weeks within the walls of a "retreat" than I could in the world outside. My one desire was to write, write, write. My fingers itched for a pen. My desire to write was, I imagine, as irresistible as is the desire of a drunkard for his dram. And the act of writing resulted in an intoxicating pleasure composed of a mingling of emotions that defies analysis.

That I should so calmly, almost eagerly, enter where devils might fear to tread may surprise the reader who already has been informed of the cruel treatment I had formerly received there. I feared nothing, for I knew all. Having seen the worst, I knew how to avoid the pitfalls into which, during my first experience at that hospital, I had fallen or deliberately walked. I was confident that I should suffer no abuse or injustice so long as the doctors in charge should live up to their agreement and treat me with unvarying fairness. This they did, and my quick recovery and subsequent discharge may be attributed partly to this cause. The assistant physicians who had come in contact with me during my first experience in this hospital were no longer there. They had resigned some months earlier, shortly after the death of the former superintendent. Thus it was that I started with a clean record, free from those prejudices which so often affect the judgment of a hospital physician who has treated a mental patient at his worst.

⚓XXX⚓

On more than one occasion my chameleonlike temperament has enabled me to adjust myself to new conditions, but never has it served me better than it did at the time of which I write. A free man on New Year's Day, enjoying the pleasures of a congenial club life, four days later I found myself again under the lock and key of an institution for the insane. Never had I enjoyed life in New York more than during those first days of that new year. To suffer so rude a change was, indeed, enough to arouse a feeling of discontent, if not despair; yet, aside from the momentary initial shock, my contentment was in no degree diminished. I can say with truth that I was as complacent the very moment I recrossed the threshold of that "retreat" as I had been when crossing and recrossing at will the threshold of my club.

Of everything I thought and did during the interesting weeks which followed, I have a complete record. The moment I accepted the inevitable, I determined to spend my time to good advantage. Knowing from experience that I must observe my own case, if I was to have any detailed record of it, I provided myself in advance with notebooks. In these I recorded, I might almost say, my every thought and action. The sane part of me, which fortunately was dominant, subjected its temporarily un-ruly part to a sort of scientific scrutiny and surveillance. From morning till night I dogged the steps of my restless body and my more restless imagination. I observed the physical and mental symptoms which I knew were characteristic of elation. An exquisite light-heartedness, an exalted sense of well-being, my pulse, my weight, my appetite—all these I observed and recorded with a care that would have put to the blush a majority of the doctors in charge of mental cases in institutions.

But this record of symptoms, though minute, was vague compared to my reckless analysis of my emotions. With a lack of reserve characteristic of my mood, I described the joy of living, which, for the most part, then consisted in the joy of writing. And even now, when I reread my record, I feel that I cannot overstate the pleasure I found in surrendering myself completely to that controlling impulse. The excellence of my composition seemed to me beyond criticism. And, as to one in a state of elation, things are pretty much as they seem, I was able to experience the subtle delights which, I fancy, thrill the soul of a master. During this month of elation I wrote words enough to fill a book nearly as large as this one. Having found that each filling of my fountain pen was sufficient for the writing of about twenty-eight hundred words, I kept a record of the number of times I filled it. This minute calculation I carried to an extreme. If I wrote for fifty-nine minutes, and then read for seventeen, those facts I recorded. Thus, in my diary and out of it, I wrote and wrote until the tips of my thumb and forefinger grew numb. As this numbness increased and general weariness of the hand set in, there came a gradual flagging of my creative impulse until a very normal unproductivity supervened.

The reader may well wonder in what my so-called insanity at this time consisted. Had I any of those impracticable delusions which had characterized my former period of elation? No, not one—unless an unreasonable haste to achieve my ambitions may be counted a delusion. My attention simply focussed itself on my project. All other considerations seemed of little moment. My interest in business waned to the vanishing point.

Yet one thing should be noted: I did deliberately devote many hours to the consideration of business affairs. Realizing that one way to overcome an absorbing impulse is to divide attention, I wrote a brief of the arguments I had often used when talking with bankers. In this way I was able to convince the doctors that my intense interest in literature and reform would soon spend itself.

A consuming desire to effect reforms had been the determining factor when I calmly weighed the situation with a view to making the best possible use of my impulse to write. The events of the immediate past had convinced me that I could not hope to interest people of wealth and influence in my humanitarian project until I had some definite plan to submit for their leisurely consideration. Further, I had discovered that an attempt to approach them directly disturbed my relatives and friends, who had not yet learned to dissociate present intentions from past performances. I had, therefore, determined to drill myself in the art of composition to the end that I might write a story of my life which would merit publication. I felt that such a book, once written, would do its own work, regardless of my subsequent fortunes. Other books had spoken even from the grave; why should not my book so speak—if necessary?

With this thought in mind I began not only to read and write, but to test my impulse in order that I might discover if it were a part of my very being, an abnormal impulse, or a mere whim. I reasoned that to compare my own feelings toward literature, and my emotions experienced in the heat of composition, with the recorded feelings of successful men of letters, would give me a clue to the truth on this question. At this time I read several books that could have served as a basis for my deductions, but only one of them did I have time to analyze and note in my diary. That one was, "Wit and Wisdom of the Earl of Beaconsfield." The following passages from the pen of Disraeli I transcribed in my diary with occasional comment.

"Remember who you are, and also that it is your duty to excel. Providence has given you a great lot. Think ever that you are born to perform great duties." This I interpreted in much the same spirit that I had interpreted the 45th Psalm on an earlier occasion.

"It was that noble ambition, the highest and best, that must be born in the heart, and organized in the brain, which will not let a man be content unless his intellectual power is recognized by his race, and desires that it should contribute to their welfare."

"Authors—the creators of opinion."

"What appear to be calamities are often the sources of fortune."

"Change is inevitable in a progressive country. Change is constant." ("Then why," was my recorded comment, "cannot the changes I propose to bring about, be brought about?")

"The author is, as we must ever remember, of peculiar organization. He is a being born with a predisposition which with him is irresistible, the bent of which he cannot in any way avoid, whether it directs him to the abstruse researches of erudition or induces him to mount into the fervid and turbulent atmosphere of imagination."

"This," I wrote (the day after arriving at the hospital) "is a fair diagnosis of my case as it stands today, assuming of course, that an author is one who loves to write, and can write with ease, even though what he says may have no literary value. My past proves that my organization is a peculiar one. I have for years (two and a half) had a desire to achieve success along literary lines. I believe that, feeling as I do today, nothing can prevent my writing. If I had to make a choice at once between a sure success in the business career ahead of me and doubtful success in the field of literature, I would willingly, yes confidently, choose the latter. I have read many a time about successful writers who learned how to write, and by dint of hard work ground out their ideas. If these men could succeed, why should not a man who is in danger of being ground up by an excess of ideas and imagination succeed, when he seems able to put those ideas into fairly intelligible English? He should and will succeed."

Therefore, without delay, I began the course of experiment and practice which culminated within a few months in the first draft of my story. Wise enough to realize the advantages of a situation free from the annoying interruptions of the workaday world, I enjoyed a degree of liberty seldom experienced by those in possession of complete legal liberty and its attendant obligations. When I wished to read, write, talk, walk, sleep, or eat, I did the thing I wished. I went to the theatre when the spirit moved me to do so, accompanied, of course, by an attendant, who on such occasions played the rôle of chum.

Friends called to see me and, at their suggestion or mine, invited me to dinner outside the walls of my "cloister." At one of these dinners an incident occurred which throws a clear light on my condition at the time. The friend, whose willing prisoner I was, had invited a common friend to join the party. The latter had not heard of my recent commitment. At my suggestion, he who shared my secret had agreed not to refer to it unless I first broached the subject. There was nothing strange in the fact that we three should meet. Just such impromptu celebrations had before occurred among us. We dined, and, as friends will, indulged in that exchange of thoughts which bespeaks intimacy. During our talk, I so shaped the conversation that the possibility of a recurrence of my mental illness was discussed. The uninformed friend derided the idea.

"Then, if I were to tell you," I remarked, "that I am at this moment supposedly insane—at least not normal—and that when I leave you tonight I shall go direct to the very hospital where I was formerly confined, there to remain until the doctors pronounce me fit for freedom, what would you say?"

"I should say that you are a choice sort of liar," he retorted.

This genial insult I swallowed with gratification. It was, in truth, a timely and encouraging compliment, the force of which its author failed to appreciate until my host had corroborated my statements.

If I could so favorably impress an intimate friend at a time when I was elated, it is not surprising that I should subsequently hold an interview with a comparative stranger—the cashier of a local bank—without betraying my state of mind. As business interviews go, this was in a class by itself. While my attendant stood guard at the door, I, an enrolled inmate of a hospital for the insane, entered the banking room and talked with a level-headed banker. And that interview was not without effect in subsequent negotiations which led to the closing of a contract amounting to one hundred and fifty thousand dollars.

The very day I re-entered the hospital I stopped on the way at a local hotel and procured some of the hostelry's stationery. By using this in the writing of personal and business letters I managed to conceal my condition and my whereabouts from all except near relatives and a few intimate friends who shared the secret. I quite enjoyed leading this legitimate double life. The situation appealed (not in vain) to my sense of humor. Many a smile did I indulge in when I closed a letter with such ambiguous phrases as the following: "Matters of importance necessitate my remaining where I am for an indefinite period." . . . "A situation has recently arisen which will delay my intended trip South. As soon as I have closed a certain contract (having in mind my contract to re-establish my sanity) I shall again take to the road." To this day few friends or acquaintances know that I was in semi-exile during the month of January, 1905. My desire to suppress the fact was not due, as already intimated, to any sensitiveness regarding the subject of insanity. What afterwards justified my course was that on regaining my freedom I was able, without embarrassment, again to take up my work. Within a month of my voluntary commitment, that is, in February, I started on a business trip through the Central West and South, where I remained until the following July. During those months I felt perfectly well, and have remained in excellent health ever since.

This second interruption of my career came at a time and in a manner to furnish me with strong arguments wherewith to support my contention that so-called madmen are too often man-made, and that he who is potentially mad may keep a saving grip on his own reason if he is fortunate enough to receive that kindly and intelligent treatment to which one on the brink of mental chaos is entitled. Though during this second period of elation I was never in a mood so reckless as that which obtained immediately after my recovery from depression in August, 1902, I was at least so excitable that, had those in authority attempted to impose upon me, I should have thrown discretion to the winds. To them, indeed, I frankly reiterated a terse dictum which I had coined during my first period of elation. "Just press the button of Injustice," I said, "and I'll do the rest!" This I meant, for fear of punishment does not restrain a man in the dare-devil grip of elation.

What fostered my self-control was a sense of gratitude. The doctors and attendants treated me as a gentleman. Therefore it was not difficult to prove myself one. My every whim was at least considered with a politeness which enabled me to accept a denial with a highly sane equanimity. Aside from mild tonics I took no other medicine than that most beneficial sort which inheres in kindness. The feeling that, though a prisoner, I could still command obligations from others led me to recognize my own reciprocal obligations, and was a constant source of delight. The doctors, by proving their title to that confidence which I tentatively gave them upon re-entering the institution, had no difficulty in convincing me that a temporary curtailment of some privileges was for my own good. They all evinced a consistent desire to trust me. In return I trusted them.

∝XXXI∝

On leaving the hospital and resuming my travels, I felt sure that any one of several magazines or newspapers would willingly have had me conduct my campaign under its nervously commercial auspices; but a flash-in-the-pan method did not appeal to me. Those noxious growths, Incompetence, Abuse, and Injustice, had not only to be cut down, but rooted out. Therefore, I clung to my determination to write a book—an instrument of attack which, if it cuts and sears at all, does so as long as the need exists. Inasmuch as I knew that I still had to learn how to write, I approached my task with deliberation. I planned to do two things: first, to crystallize my thoughts by discussion—telling the story of my life whenever in my travels I should meet any person who inspired my confidence; second, while the subject matter of my book was shaping itself in my mind, to drill myself by carrying on a letter-writing campaign. Both of these things I did—as certain indulgent friends who bore the brunt of my spoken and written discourse can certify. I feared the less to be dubbed a bore, and I hesitated the less, perhaps, to impose upon good-nature, because of my firm conviction that one in a position to help the many was himself entitled to the help of the few.

I wrote scores of letters of great length. I cared little if some of my friends should conclude that I had been born a century too late; for, without them as confidants, I must write with no more inspiring object in view than the wastebasket. Indeed, I

191

found it difficult to compose without keeping before me the image of a friend. Having stipulated that every letter should be returned upon demand, I wrote without reserve—my imagination had free rein. I wrote as I thought, and I thought as I pleased. The result was that within six months I found myself writing with a facility which hitherto had obtained only during elation. At first I was suspicious of this new-found and apparently permanent ease of expression—so suspicious that I set about diagnosing my symptoms. My self-examination convinced me that I was, in fact, quite normal. I had no irresistible desire to write, nor was there any suggestion of that exalted, or (technically speaking) euphoric, lightheartedness which characterizes elation. Further, after a prolonged period of composition, I experienced a comforting sense of exhaustion which I had not known while elated. I therefore concluded—and rightly—that my unwonted facility was the product of practice. At last I found myself able to conceive an idea and immediately transfer it to paper effectively.

In July, 1905, I came to the conclusion that the time for beginning my book was at hand. Nevertheless, I found it difficult to set a definite date. About this time I so arranged my itinerary that I was able to enjoy two summer—though stormy —nights and a day at the Summit House on Mount Washington. What better, thought I, than to begin my book on a plane so high as to be appropriate to this noble summit? I therefore began to compose a dedication. "To Humanity" was as far as I got. There the Muse forsook me.

But, returning to earth and going about my business, I soon again found myself in the midst of inspiring natural surroundings—the Berkshire Hills. At this juncture Man came to the assistance of Nature, and perhaps with an unconsciousness equal to her own. It was a chance remark made by an eminent man that aroused my subconscious literary personality to irresistible action. I had long wished to discuss my project with a man of great reputation, and if the reputation were international, so much the better. I desired the unbiased opinion of a judicial mind. Opportunely, I learned that the Hon. Joseph H. Choate was then at his summer residence at Stockbridge, Massachusetts. Mr. Choate had never heard of me and I had no letter of introduction. The exigencies of the occasion, however, demanded that I conjure one up, so I wrote my own letter of introduction and sent it:

> RED LION INN,
> STOCKBRIDGE, MASS.
> August 18, 1906.

HON. JOSEPH H. CHOATE,
Stockbridge, Massachusetts.

DEAR SIR:

Though I might present myself at your door, armed with one of society's unfair skeleton-keys—a letter of introduction— I prefer to approach you as I now do: simply as a young man who honestly feels entitled to at least five minutes of your time, and as many minutes more as you care to grant because of your interest in the subject to be discussed.

I look to you at this time for your opinion as to the value of some ideas of mine, and the feasibility of certain schemes based on them.

A few months ago I talked with President Hadley of Yale, and briefly outlined my plans. He admitted that many of them seemed feasible and would, if carried out, add much to the sum-total of human happiness. His only criticism was that they were "too comprehensive."

Not until I have staggered an imagination of the highest type will I admit that I am trying to do too much. Should you refuse to see me, believe me when I tell you that you will still be, as you are at this moment, the unconscious possessor of my sincere respect.

Business engagements necessitate my leaving here early on Monday next. Should you care to communicate with me, word sent in care of this hotel will reach me promptly.

Yours very truly,
CLIFFORD W. BEERS.

Within an hour I had received a reply, in which Mr. Choate said that he would see me at his home at ten o'clock the next morning.

At the appointed time, the door, whose lock I had picked with a pen, opened before me and I was ushered into the presence of Mr. Choate. He was graciousness itself—but pointed significantly at a heap of unanswered letters lying before him. I took the hint and within ten minutes briefly outlined my plans. After pronouncing my project a "commendable one," Mr. Choate offered the suggestion that produced results. "If you will submit your ideas in writing," he said, "I shall be glad to read your manuscript and assist you in any way I can. To consider fully your scheme would require several hours, and busy men cannot very well give you so much time. What they can do is to read your manuscript during their leisure moments."

Thus it was that Mr. Choate, by granting the interview, contributed to an earlier realization of my purposes. One week later I began the composition of this book. My action was unpremeditated, as my quitting Boston for less attractive Worcester proves. That very day, finding myself with a day and a half of leisure before me, I decided to tempt the Muse and compel myself to prove that my pen was, in truth, "the tongue of a ready writer." A stranger in the city, I went to a school of stenography and there secured the services of a young man who, though inexperienced in his art, was more skilled in catching thoughts as they took wing than I was at that time in the art of setting them free. Except in the writing of one or two conventional business letters, never before had I dictated to a stenographer. After I had startled him into an attentive mood by briefly outlining my past career and present purpose, I worked without any definite plan or brief, or reference to data. My narrative was therefore digressive and only roughly chronological. But it served to get my material in front of me for future shaping. At this task I hammered away three or four hours a day for a period of five weeks.

It so happened that Mr. Choate arrived at the same hotel on the day I took up my abode there, so that some of the toil he had inspired went on in his proximity, if not in his presence. I carefully kept out of his sight, however, lest he should think me a "crank" on the subject of reform, bent on persecuting his leisure.

As the work progressed my facility increased. In fact, I soon called in an additional stenographer to help in the snaring of my thoughts. This excessive productivity caused me to pause and again diagnose my condition. I could not fail now to recognize in myself symptoms hardly distinguishable from those which had obtained eight months earlier when it had been deemed expedient temporarily to restrict my freedom. But I had grown wise in adversity. Rather than interrupt my manuscript short of completion I decided to avail myself of a vacation that was due, and remain outside my native State—this so that well-meaning but perhaps over-zealous relatives might be spared unnecessary anxiety, and I myself be spared possible unwarranted restrictions. I was by no means certain as to the degree of mental excitement that would result from such continuous mental application; nor did I much care, so long as I accomplished my task. However, as I knew that "possession is nine points of the law," I decided to maintain my advantage by remaining in my literary fortress. And my resolve was further strengthened by certain cherished sentiments expressed by John

Stuart Mill in his essay "On Liberty," which I had read and re-read with an interest born of experience.

At last the first draft of the greater part of my story was completed. After a timely remittance (for, in strict accordance with the traditions of the craft, I had exhausted my financial resources) I started for home with a sigh of relief. For months I had been under the burden of a conscious obligation. My memory, stored with information which, if rightly used, could, I believed, brighten and even save unhappy lives, was to me as a basket of eggs which it was my duty to balance on a head whose poise was supposed to be none too certain. One by one, during the preceding five weeks, I had gently lifted my thoughts from their resting-place, until a large part of my burden had been so shifted as to admit of its being imposed upon the public conscience.

After I had lived over again the trials and the tortures of my unhappiest years—which was of course necessary in ploughing and harrowing a memory happily retentive—the completion of this first draft left me exhausted. But after a trip to New York, whither I went to convince my employers that I should be granted a further leave-of-absence, I resumed work. The ground for this added favor was that my manuscript was too crude to submit to any but intimate acquaintances. Knowing, perhaps, that a business man with a literary bee buzzing in his ear is, for the time, no business man at all, my employers readily agreed that I should do as I pleased during the month of October. They also believed me entitled to the favor, recognizing the force of my belief that I had a high obligation to discharge.

It was under the family rooftree that I now set up my literary shop. Nine months earlier an unwonted interest in literature and reform had sent me to an institution. That I should now in my own home be able to work out my destiny without unduly disturbing the peace of mind of relatives was a considerable satisfaction. In the very room where, during June, 1900, my reason had set out for an unknown goal, I redictated my account of that reason's experiences.

My leave-of-absence ended, I resumed my travels eagerly; for I wished to cool my brain by daily contact with the more prosaic minds of men of business. I went South. For a time I banished all thoughts of my book and project. But after some months of this change of occupation, which I thoroughly enjoyed, I found leisure in the course of wide travels to take up the work of elaboration and revision. A presentable draft of my story being finally prepared, I began to submit it to all sorts and conditions of minds (in accordance with Mill's dictum that only in that way can the truth be obtained). In my quest for criticism and advice, I fortunately decided to submit my manuscript to Professor William James of Harvard University, the most eminent of American psychologists and a masterful writer, who was then living. He expressed interest in my project; put my manuscript with others on his desk—but was somewhat reserved when it came to promising to read my story. He said it might be months before he could find time to do so. Within a fortnight, however, I received from him a characteristic letter. To me it came as a rescuing sun, after a period of groping about for an authoritative opinion that should put scoffers to flight. The letter read as follows:

95 IRVING ST., CAMBRIDGE, MASS.
July 1, 1906.

DEAR MR. BEERS:

Having at last "got round" to your MS., I have read it with very great interest and admiration for both its style and its temper. I hope you will finish it and publish it. It is the best written out "case" that I have seen; and you no doubt have put your finger on the weak spots of our treatment of the insane, and suggested the right line of remedy. I have long thought that if I were a millionaire, with money to leave for public purposes, I should endow "Insanity" exclusively.

You were doubtless a pretty intolerable character when the maniacal condition came on and you were bossing the universe. Not only ordinary "tact," but a genius for diplomacy must have been needed for avoiding rows with you; but you certainly were wrongly treated nevertheless; and the spiteful Assistant M.D. at —— deserves to have his name published. Your report is full of instructiveness for doctors and attendants alike.

The most striking thing in it to my mind is the sudden conversion of you from a delusional subject to a maniacal one—how the whole delusional system disintegrated the moment one pin was drawn out by your proving your brother to be genuine. I never heard of so rapid a change in a mental system.

You speak of rewriting. Don't you do it. You can hardly improve your book. I shall keep the MS. a week longer as I wish to impart it to a friend.

Sincerely yours,
WM. JAMES.

Though Mr. James paid me the compliment of advising me not to rewrite my original manuscript, I did revise it quite thoroughly before publication. When my book was about to go to press for the first time and since its reception by the public was problematical, I asked permission to publish the letter already quoted. In reply, Mr. James sent the following letter, also for publication:

95 IRVING ST., CAMBRIDGE, MASS.
November 10, 1907.

DEAR MR. BEERS:

You are welcome to use the letter I wrote to you (on July 1, 1906) after reading the first part of your MS. in any way your judgment prompts, whether as preface, advertisement, or anything else. Reading the rest of it only heightens its importance in my eyes. In style, in temper, in good taste, it is irreproachable. As for contents, it is fit to remain in literature as a classic account "from within" of an insane person's psychology.

The book ought to go far toward helping along that terribly needed reform, the amelioration of the lot of the insane of our country, for the Auxiliary Society which you propose is feasible (as numerous examples in other fields show), and ought to work important effects on the whole situation.

You have handled a difficult theme with great skill, and produced a narrative of absorbing interest to scientist as well as layman. It reads like fiction, but it is not fiction; and this I state emphatically, knowing how prone the uninitiated are to doubt the truthfulness of descriptions of abnormal mental processes.

With best wishes for the success of the book and the plan, both of which, I hope, will prove epoch-making, I remain,

Sincerely yours,
WM. JAMES

Several times in my narrative, I have said that the seemingly unkind fate that robbed me of several probably happy and healthful years had hidden within it compensations which have offset the sufferings and the loss of those years. Not the least of the compensations has been the many letters sent to me by eminent men and women, who, having achieved results in their own work, are ever responsive to the efforts of anyone trying to reach a difficult objective. Of all the encouraging opinions I have ever received, one has its own niche in my memory. It came from William James a few months before his death, and will ever be an inspiration to me. Let my excuse for revealing so complimentary a letter be that it justifies the hopes and aspirations expressed in the course of my narrative, and shows them to be well on the way to accomplishment.

95 IRVING ST., CAMBRIDGE,
January 17, 1910.

DEAR BEERS:

Your exegesis of my farewell in my last note to you was erroneous, but I am glad it occurred, because it brought me to the extreme gratification of your letter of yesterday.

You are the most responsive and recognizant of human beings, my dear Beers, and it "sets me up immensely" to be treated by a practical man on practical grounds as you treat me. I inhabit such a realm of abstractions that I only get credit for what I do in that spectral empire; but you are not only a moral idealist and philanthropic enthusiast (and good fellow!), but a tip-top man of business in addition; and to have actually done anything that the like of you can regard as having helped him is an unwonted ground with me for self-gratulation. I think that your tenacity of purpose, foresight, tact, temper, discretion and patience, are beyond all praise, and I esteem it an honor to have been in any degree associated with you. Your name will loom big hereafter, for your movement must prosper, but mine will not survive unless some other kind of effort of mine saves it.

I am exceedingly glad of what you say of the Connecticut Society. May it prosper abundantly!

I thank you for your affectionate words which I return with interest and remain, for I trust many years of this life,

Yours faithfully,
WM. JAMES.

At this point, rather than in the dusty corners of the usual preface, I wish to express my obligation to Herbert Wescott Fisher, whom I knew at school. It was he who led me to see my need of technical training, neglected in earlier years. To be exact, however, I must confess that I read rather than studied rhetoric. Close application to its rules served only to discourage me, so I but lazily skimmed the pages of the works which he recommended. But my friend did more than direct me to sources. He proved to be the kindly mean between the two extremes of stranger and intimate. I was a prophet not without honor in his eyes. Upon an embarrassing wealth of material he brought to bear his practical knowledge of the workmanship of writing; and my drafting of the later parts and subsequent revisions has been so improved by the practice received under his scrupulous direction that he has had little fault to find with them. My debt to him is almost beyond repayment.

Nothing would please me more than to express specifically my indebtedness to many others who have assisted me in the preparation of my work. But, aside from calling attention to the fact that physicians connected with the State Hospital and with the private institution referred to—the one not run for profit—exhibited rare magnanimity (even going so far as to write letters which helped me in my work), and, further, acknowledging anonymously (the list is too long for explicit mention) the invaluable advice given me by psychiatrists who have enabled me to make my work authoritative, I must be content to indite an all-embracing acknowledgment. Therefore, and with distinct pleasure, I wish to say that the active encouragement of casual, but trusted acquaintances, the inspiring indifference of unconvinced intimates, and the kindly scepticism of indulgent relatives, who, perforce, could do naught but obey an immutable law of blood-related minds—all these influences have conspired to render more sure the accomplishment of my heart's desire.

↔XXXII↔

"My heart's desire" is a true phrase. Since 1900, when my own breakdown occurred, not fewer than one million men and women in the United States alone have for like causes had to seek treatment in institutions, thousands of others have been treated outside of institutions, while other thousands have received no treatment at all. Yet, to use the words of one of our most conservative and best informed psychiatrists, "No less than half of the enormous toll which mental disease takes from the youth of this country can be prevented by the application, largely in childhood, of information and practical resources now available."

Elsewhere is an account of how my plan broadened from reform to cure, from cure to prevention,—how far, with the co-operation of some of this country's ablest specialists and most generous philanthropists, it has been realized, nationally and internationally, through the new form of social mechanism known as societies, committees, leagues or associations for mental hygiene.

More fundamental, however, than any technical reform, cure, or prevention—indeed, a condition precedent to all these —is a changed spiritual attitude toward the insane. They are still human: they love and hate, and have a sense of humor. The worst are usually responsive to kindness. In not a few cases their gratitude is livelier than that of normal men and women.

Any person who has worked among the insane, and done his duty by them, can testify to cases in point; and even casual observers have noted the fact that the insane are oftentimes appreciative. Consider the experience of Thackeray, as related by himself in "Vanity Fair" (Chapter LVII). "I recollect," he writes, "seeing, years ago, at the prison for idiots and madmen, at Bicêtre, near Paris, a poor wretch bent down under the bondage of his imprisonment and his personal infirmity, to whom one of our party gave a halfpennyworth of snuff in a cornet or 'screw' of paper. The kindness was too much . . . He cried in an anguish of delight and gratitude; if anybody gave you and me a thousand a year, or saved our lives, we could not be so affected."

A striking exhibition of fine feeling on the part of a patient was brought to my attention by an assistant physician whom I met while visiting a State Hospital in Massachusetts. It seems that the woman in question had, at her worst, caused an endless amount of annoyance by indulging in mischievous acts which seemed to verge on malice. At that time, therefore, no observer would have credited her with the exquisite sensibility she so signally displayed when she had become convalescent and was granted a parole which permitted her to walk at will about the hospital grounds. After one of these walks, taken in the early spring, she rushed up to my informant and, with childlike simplicity, told him of the thrill of delight she had experienced in discovering the first flower of the year in full bloom—a dandelion, which, with characteristic audacity, had risked its life by braving the elements of an uncertain season.

"Did you pick it?" asked the doctor.

"I stooped to do so," said the patient; "then I thought of the pleasure the sight of it had given me—so I left it, hoping that someone else would discover it and enjoy its beauty as I did."

Thus it was that a woman, while still insane, unconsciously exhibited perhaps finer feeling than did Ruskin, Tennyson, and

Patmore on an occasion the occurrence of which is vouched for by Mr. Julian Hawthorne. These three masters, out for a walk one chilly afternoon in late autumn, discovered a belated violet bravely putting forth from the shelter of a mossy stone. Not until these worthies had got down on all fours and done ceremonious homage to the flower did they resume their walk. Suddenly Ruskin halted and, planting his cane in the ground, exclaimed, "I don't believe, Alfred—Coventry, I don't believe that there are in all England three men besides ourselves who, after finding a violet at this time of year, would have had forbearance and fine feeling enough to refrain from plucking it."

The reader may judge whether the unconscious display of feeling by the obscure inmate of a hospital for the insane was not finer than the self-conscious raptures of these three men of worldwide reputation.

Is it not, then, an atrocious anomaly that the treatment often meted out to insane persons is the very treatment which would deprive some sane persons of their reason? Miners and shepherds who penetrate the mountain fastnesses sometimes become mentally unbalanced as a result of prolonged loneliness. But they usually know enough to return to civilization when they find themselves beginning to be affected with hallucinations. Delay means death. Contact with sane people, if not too long postponed, means an almost immediate restoration to normality. This is an illuminating fact. Inasmuch as patients cannot usually be set free to absorb, as it were, sanity in the community, it is the duty of those entrusted with their care to treat them with the utmost tenderness and consideration.

"After all," said a psychiatrist who had devoted a long life to work among the insane, both as an assistant physician and later as superintendent at various private and public hospitals, "what the insane most need is a *friend!*"

These words, spoken to me, came with a certain startling freshness. And yet it was the sublime and healing power of this same love which received its most signal demonstration two thousand years ago at the hand of one who restored to reason and his home that man of Scripture "who had his dwelling among the tombs; and no man could bind him, no, not with chains: Because that he had been often bound with fetters and chains, and the chains had been plucked asunder by him, and the fetters broken in pieces; neither could any man tame him. And always, night and day, he was in the mountains, and in the tombs, crying, and cutting himself with stones. But when he saw Jesus afar off, he ran and worshipped him, And cried with a loud voice, and said, What have I to do with Thee, Jesus, Thou Son of the Most High God? I adjure Thee by God, that Thou torment me not."

Bibliographical Note

For this edition, the text of *A Mind That Found Itself* has been completely reset from the fifth edition, first issued in 1921. Beers prepared the fifth edition himself, making minor changes in wording and cutting approximately forty pages of what had appeared as Part II of the first edition (in these pages, Beers had reiterated and expanded his recommendations for more humane and individualized medical care for patients in mental institutions). The introductory letters from William James and Booth Tarkington and the supplementary material on the mental hygiene movement that Beers appended to the fifth edition have also been omitted here.